Epilepsy

Questions and Answers

2ND EDITION

D1244685

Y M HART, MA, MD, FRCP
Department of Neurology, John Radcliffe Hospital, Oxford

J W SANDER, MD, PhD, FRCP
Department of Clinical and Experimental Epilepsy, UCL Institute of Neurology, London
and SEIN–Epilepsy Institutes of the Netherlands Foundation – Heemstede, The Netherlands

m rit
PUBLISHING
INTERNATIONAL

Cover Design and Artwork by:

SMK Design

m e rit
PUBLISHING
INTERNATIONAL

Epilepsy

Questions and Answers

2ND EDITION

MERIT PUBLISHING INTERNATIONAL

European address:
50 Highpoint, Heath Road
Weybridge, Surrey KT13 8TP
England

Tel: (44) (0) 1932 844526

Email: merituk@aol.com

North American address:
1095 Jupiter Park Drive,
Suite 7, Jupiter, FL 33458
USA

Tel: 561 697 1116

Email: meritpi@aol.com

Web: www.meritpublishing.com

ISBN: 978 1 873413 87 6

PUBLISHING
INTERNATIONAL

CONTENTS

Epilepsy

Questions and Answers

2ND EDITION

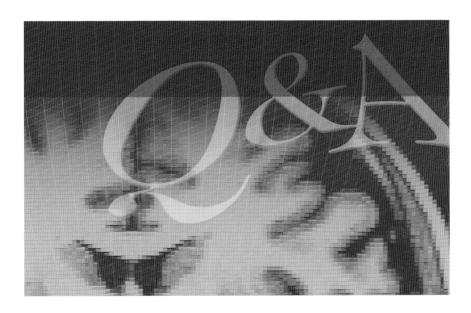

Y M HART, MA, MD, FRCP

Department of Neurology, John Radcliffe Hospital, Oxford

J W SANDER, MD, PhD, FRCP

Department of Clinical and Experimental Epilepsy, UCL Institute of Neurology, London
and SEIN–Epilepsy Institutes of the Netherlands Foundation – Heemstede, The Netherlands

merit

PUBLISHING
INTERNATIONAL

INTRODUCTION

Epilepsy is a common medical condition, with a lifetime incidence estimated at 2-5%. The majority of people diagnosed as having epilepsy have only a few seizures, usually each lasting only minutes, and yet the implications of the diagnosis are often considerable, particularly in the areas of employment, education and leisure. Apart from the limitations imposed by the risk of a seizure itself, epilepsy has long been beset by myths and negative conceptions, even among the medical profession, which until recently considered epilepsy to be a lifelong condition with a uniformly poor prognosis.

This is the second edition of this practical guide to epilepsy. Like the first edition, it has been written for general physicians, general practitioners, epilepsy nurses, neurologists in training, and medical students, to provide a concise core of background information on the nature, causes, and treatment of epilepsy, and to supply answers to some of the questions most commonly asked by patients regarding these issues. The format is similar to that of the first edition but the book has been completely updated. It is not intended to supplant standard textbooks of epilepsy, which are recommended for further reading and reference. A basic knowledge of neuroanatomy and physiology has been assumed.

The book is divided into thirteen chapters. The first five describe the epidemiology, nature and characteristics of epilepsy and other seizure disorders. Chapter six addresses the question of the diagnosis of epilepsy and the investigations which may be required to confirm diagnosis, classify the type of epilepsy and evaluate the underlying cause. The next two chapters deal with the types of medical and surgical treatment currently available and their indications. Women with epilepsy pose specific problems such as the management of epilepsy during pregnancy, the issue of teratogenicity associated with antiepileptic drugs, menstruation and contraception, and these are dealt with in chapter nine. The psychiatric aspects of epilepsy and the issues of genetic counseling in epilepsy are addressed in the next two chapters. Issues of leisure and work are dealt with in Chapter 12, while the final chapter is a selection of questions frequently asked by people with epilepsy. A reading list and the web addresses of epilepsy organizations worldwide are also provided in the appendices.

Epilepsy poses a number of peculiar problems. Unlike most ailments, it is episodic: in between seizures, physical examination and laboratory investigation of patients may be perfectly normal. The diagnosis is, therefore, essentially clinical, relying on the patient's account and those of eye-witnesses, and it may be difficult to differentiate seizures from the myriad of other episodic conditions capable of causing transient impairment of consciousness or other symptoms. Because of the potential impact on the patient's life, however, it is imperative that the correct diagnosis is reached, and that optimum treatment and advice are given.

Although we have tried to ensure that the information contained in this book, particularly pertaining to drugs, is accurate, drug information may change from time to time and clinicians are strongly advised to consult manufacturers' information sheets and national prescribing guidelines where available before prescribing drugs.

CHAPTER 1

What is epilepsy?

Epilepsy is one of the most common neurological conditions affecting at any given time between 0.5% and 1.0% of the general population in developed countries. It is also one of the oldest recorded medical conditions, having been accurately described by Hippocrates more than 2000 years ago. The word "epilepsy" is derived from a Greek term, meaning to possess, to take hold of, to grab or to seize. To the ancient Greeks, epilepsy was a miraculous phenomenon; they considered that only the gods could knock someone down, strip their reason, make their body thrash around uncontrollably, and afterwards bring them around without apparent ill-effect.

A common neurological condition

The first modern definition of epilepsy was given by Hughlings Jackson in the second half of the 19th century. He defined it as *"the occasional, sudden, excessive, rapid and local discharge of grey matter"*, and this definition is among those used today, although it should be pointed out that discharges detected electrographically are not generally considered to be clinical seizures unless they are accompanied by changes which can be detected either by the patient or an observer. An operational definition of epilepsy often used currently is *"the occurrence of transient paroxysms of excessive or uncontrolled discharges of neurons, which may be caused by a number of different etiologies, leading to epileptic seizures"*. The actual form which an epileptic seizure takes, depends on the location of the initial epileptic discharge and its spread.

Excessive discharges of neurons

It is necessary for seizures to be recurrent and unprovoked to constitute epilepsy: by definition a single attack is not considered sufficient to make this diagnosis, even though most people having one seizure will have further attacks. Epileptic seizures occurring only in association with precipitants or trigger factors are termed acute symptomatic or situation-related seizures: even if recurrent, they are not usually considered to be "epilepsy". Such precipitants include fever in young children, sleep deprivation, eclampsia, metabolic imbalance, alcohol or drug abuse, acute head trauma (concussive seizures), and the consumption of known epileptogenic drugs.

It should be stressed that unprovoked epileptic seizures are a symptom of a condition, rather than a single well-defined illness. The term "epilepsy" is thus loosely applied to a number of seizure disorders that have in common only a tendency for the patient to have recurrent epileptic attacks, and it has been argued that "the epilepsies" is a more appropriate term than "epilepsy". There are a number of conditions presenting with epileptic seizures, which are associated with well-defined clinical and electrophysiological characteristics that allow them to be grouped into specific epileptic syndromes, but a large number of people developing seizures cannot be grouped into such categories.

Seizures are a symptom of a brain condition

1.1   What is an epileptic seizure?

An epileptic seizure (also termed "ictus" or "ictal event") *is a transient paroxysm of excessive discharges of neurons in the cerebral cortex causing an event which is discernible to the person experiencing the seizure or an observer.* The clinical manifestations of seizures may take many different forms, varying from patient to patient and reflecting the functions of the cortical tissues in which the excessive discharge arises and to which it spreads.

A discernible event

A seizure is a stereotyped event in which an individual's awareness of his surroundings may be impaired and behavior altered. Motor signs, sensory or psychic experiences, autonomic disturbances and negative neurological phenomena (such as speech arrest or loss of muscle tone) may also occur in combination or in isolation, sometimes in a progressive manner. *Epileptic seizures frequently have a sudden onset and usually cease spontaneously.* They are commonly brief, lasting from seconds to minutes, and are often followed by a period of drowsiness and confusion (the post-ictal period).

Awareness may be impaired

Sudden onset

The word seizure is also occasionally used for other transient non-epileptic events such as syncope, psychogenic attacks, night terrors and temper tantrums, and it is thus advisable to use the term "epileptic seizure" when referring to an epileptic event. *Lay people may use many different terms to describe epileptic seizures;* some of the more frequently used are fits, spells, funny turns, funny do's, attacks and blackouts.

Terms used by the public

CHAPTER 2

THE CLASSIFICATION OF EPILEPTIC SEIZURES AND SYNDROMES

2.1 How are epileptic seizures classified?

There are several ways in which epileptic seizures may be classified. These include classification by underlying etiology, by age at onset, by the topographic location of the abnormal discharge, by the clinical manifestations, by the findings on the electroencephalogram (EEG), or by the types of seizures themselves. The question of classification is controversial and there is no universal agreement as to the most appropriate method. A comprehensive five-axis classification based on seizure phenomenology and type (whether focal or generalized seizures), syndrome, etiology and associated deficits proposed by the International League Against Epilepsy (ILAE)[1] is currently being discussed. In terms of seizures, however, **the most commonly used classification of epileptic seizures is still the International Seizure Classification[2] put forward by the ILAE more than 2 decades ago.** This is based on the clinical and electroencephalographic manifestations of a seizure (Table 1). It divides epileptic seizures into two main groups according to the source of the primary epileptic discharge: those originating from localized cortical areas, the epileptic focus or foci (partial seizures) and those characterized by synchronous discharges over both hemispheres (generalized seizures). It does not take into account the background etiology or any anatomic feature. In addition, there is a group of seizures which are deemed "unclassifiable" even after extensive investigation, such as may occur in patients with infrequent and unwitnessed events.

Classification of epileptic seizures

International League Against Epilepsy

2.2 What are partial seizures?

Partial or focal seizures arise from an epileptic focus, that is, a localized region of cerebral cortex in which the excessive discharge of neurons originates. The clinical manifestations of a partial seizure depend on the position of the focus in the

Partial seizures arise from a localized region

cerebral cortex, whether the discharge remains localized or spreads, and if it spreads, the cortical pathways involved.

The most common sites of origin of epileptic seizures are the temporal lobes. Seizures arising from the frontal lobes are also not uncommon. Less frequently the site of origin of the seizure is found in the parietal or occipital regions.

Most common sites are the temporal lobes

I. **PARTIAL SEIZURES** (seizures beginning locally)

    A. Simple partial seizures (consciousness not impaired)

        1. With motor symptoms
        2. With somatosensory or special sensory symptoms
        3. With autonomic symptoms
        4. With psychic symptoms

    B. Complex partial seizures (with impairment of consciousness)

        1. Beginning as a simple partial seizure and progressing to impairment of consciousness

            a. With no other features
            b. With features as in A. 1-4
            c. With automatisms

        2. With impairment of consciousness at onset.

            a. With no other features
            b. With features as in A. 1-4
            c. With automatisms

    C. Partial seizures secondarily generalized.

II. **GENERALIZED SEIZURES** (Bilaterally symmetrical and without focal onset)

    A. 1. Absence seizures
       2. Atypical absence seizures

    B. Myoclonic seizures

    C. Clonic seizures

    D. Tonic seizures

    E. Tonic clonic seizures

    F. Atonic seizures

III. **UNCLASSIFIED EPILEPTIC SEIZURES** (inadequate or incomplete data)

Epilepsia 1981, 22:489-501

Table 1. International Classification of Epileptic Seizures.

The partial nature of the seizure and the location of the focus can often be identified from the clinical signs present either during or after the seizure. The "aura" or warning occurring prior to a seizure experienced by some persons with epilepsy usually reflects the function of that part of the cerebral cortex in which the epileptic discharge initially occurs. If the epileptic discharge remains localized it is likely that the patient will remain aware throughout the attack, as the rest of the cortex continues to function normally. If it spreads to the limbic system consciousness may be altered, and if further spread occurs a generalized tonic clonic convulsion may follow. Another sign which indicates the partial nature of a seizure is the occurrence of post-ictal focal neurological deficits. For example, a patient may experience a transient post-ictal hemiparesis (Todd's paresis), amaurosis, or aphasia. ***The EEG tracing recorded from the scalp can also sometimes be useful in identifying the location of the focus*** (Figure 1). In patients in whom the site of origin is remote from the surface electrodes, or in whom generalization occurs very quickly, however, this may not be possible. In these cases, intracranial EEG recording may be helpful if surgery is being considered.

Nature of the seizure

EEG is also useful in identification of focus

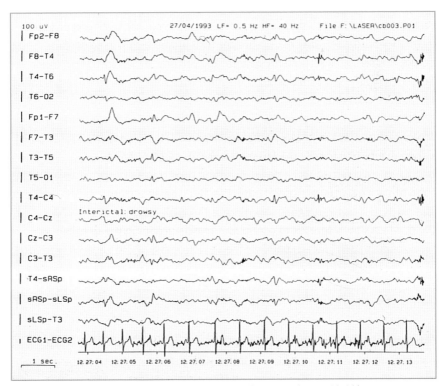

Figure 1. *EEG showing interictal focal epileptic activity. (Courtesy of Dr David Fish).*

2.3 How are partial seizures sub-divided?

Partial seizures are sub-divided into three groups: simple partial, complex partial and partial with secondary generalization.

SIMPLE PARTIAL SEIZURES

Simple partial seizures are epileptic events in which consciousness is fully preserved, and in which the discharge usually remains localized. Isolated simple partial seizures are relatively rare as they usually progress to other forms of partial seizures. Simple partial seizures are more common in persons with seizures starting late in life rather than in childhood, and almost invariably indicate the presence of a structural lesion involving the cortex. The precise clinical manifestations of a simple partial seizure depend on the cortical area in which the discharge occurs and may vary widely from patient to patient, but will usually assume the same form in one patient. Examples of such manifestations include involuntary localized motor disturbances, which may be tonic or clonic in nature, autonomic disturbances and sensory or psychic experiences. Simple partial seizures usually start suddenly and are brief, unless progression occurs. If seizure spread occurs so that consciousness is impaired, the seizure evolves into a complex partial seizure. If it progresses further and a convulsive seizure occurs, it is termed a secondarily generalized seizure. When such progression occurs, the early part of the seizure, in which consciousness is preserved, is called the aura or warning.

Consciousness is fully preserved

Motor disturbances in simple partial seizures may involve any part of the body, although most commonly the face and limbs, particularly the hands, are involved. A well-known, though rather uncommon, form of simple partial motor seizure is the "Jacksonian seizure". This starts as a clonic jerking in one part of the body, often in a hand, which slowly spreads to contiguous muscle groups in the so-called "Jacksonian march", which parallels the slow progress of the epileptic discharge along the motor cortex. Occasionally, simple partial seizures may be followed by transient weakness or even paralysis of the muscle groups involved in the seizure (Todd's paresis).

Involvement of body parts

Simple partial seizures may sometimes involve auditory, olfactory or visual hallucinations, which may be confounded with psychotic symptomatology.

In favor of an epileptic nature for hallucinations are the stereotyped nature of the attack and the fact that the patient is usually aware that the hallucinations are not real. In schizophrenia, in contrast, stereotyping of the hallucinations is absent and the patient does not have insight.

It is rather unusual for simple partial seizures to occur as the sole manifestation of epilepsy, although it may be that, because they cause little or no disability, they occur more frequently than is recognized. *Search for underlying etiology* **The development of simple partial seizures indicates the need to search for the underlying etiology, and in particular to rule out an expanding intracerebral lesion.**

COMPLEX PARTIAL SEIZURES

Complex partial seizures, one of the most common types of seizure, may have similar characteristics to simple partial seizures, but **by definition always involve an impairment of consciousness.** They are often termed "psychomotor seizures". Another term sometimes used for complex partial seizures, mainly in medical circles, is "temporal lobe epilepsy". However, it should be stressed that although *Impairment of consciousness* the majority of complex partial seizures originate in the temporal lobes, many complex partial seizures originate elsewhere, particularly in the frontal lobes.

Complex partial seizures may start as a simple partial seizure and then progress, or the patient may have alteration of consciousness from the onset. If the attack begins as a simple partial seizure, this may act as a warning (or "aura") to the patient that a seizure is about to start.

It is not uncommon for complex partial seizures to present as altered or "automatic" behavior. The patient may pluck at his or her clothes, fiddle with various objects and act in a confused manner. Lip smacking or chewing movements, grimacing, undressing and the carrying out of purposeless activities or of aimless wandering may occur *Altered or "automatic" behavior* on their own or in different combinations. Complex partial seizures are often followed by confusion in the post-ictal period; alternatively they may progress to a secondarily generalized seizure.

Automatic behavior may occur either as an ictal phenomenon or in the post-ictal period. Ictal automatisms may be either spontaneous or reactive, the former type being stereotyped, so that they usually assume the same form in each seizure. They commonly involve oroalimentary automatisms (lip-smacking, swallowing and chewing), mimetic automatisms (grimacing and other facial expressions), gestural automatisms (fiddling with clothes, undressing, scratching, rearranging objects), ambulatory automatisms (walking or running) and verbal automatisms (uttering names or phrases). Spontaneous sexual automatisms are much rarer than the above and usually involve masturbation.

Reactive automatisms are not stereotyped, but are usually determined by environmental circumstances. They generally

Determined by environmental circumstances

occur when a person has a seizure while a task is being carried out, and is able to carry on with very few outward signs of a seizure in progression. The tasks are usually simple, although on occasion more complex tasks may be performed. In the latter situation, however, an inappropriate response is more common.

SECONDARILY GENERALIZED SEIZURES

Secondarily generalized attacks are partial seizures, either simple or complex, in which the epileptic discharge spreads to both cerebral hemispheres so that a

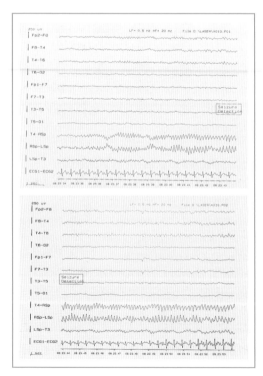

Figure 2. EEG showing progression of partial seizure originating in the right temporal lobe. (Courtesy of Dr David Fish).

generalized seizure, usually a tonic clonic convulsion, ensues. The patient may have an aura, but this is not always the case. The spread of the discharge can occur so quickly that no features of the localized onset are apparent to the patient or to an observer, and in that case only an EEG can demonstrate the partial nature of the seizure (Figure 2). On rare occasions a secondarily generalized seizure may take the form of a tonic, atonic or unilateral tonic clonic seizure.

Tonic clonic convulsion

2.4 What are generalized seizures?

Generalized seizures are characterized by the simultaneous involvement of the whole cortex at the onset of the seizure. An EEG can usually demonstrate this. Patients experiencing generalized seizures lose consciousness at the beginning of the seizure, so that there is no warning. There are various types of generalized seizures (Table 1). Among the most common generalized epileptic attacks are generalized tonic clonic seizures, absence seizures, myoclonic, tonic and atonic seizures.

Involvement of the whole cortex

GENERALIZED TONIC CLONIC SEIZURES

Generalized tonic clonic convulsions, or convulsive seizures, are common. They used to be called "grand mal" attacks, and this term is still widely used. In this type of seizure, there is no warning whatsoever, but the patient may experience a prodrome, sometimes lasting hours, of general malaise. At the onset of the seizure (the tonic phase), the patient becomes stiff, often crying out. The tongue may also be bitten during this phase. Apnea occurs, and the patient becomes cyanosed. The heart rate and blood pressure increase. The patient falls, breathing becomes labored, salivation occurs, and clonic movements, usually involving all four limbs, develop (the clonic phase). This phase consists of intermittent clonic movements involving most muscles, followed by brief periods of muscle relaxation. The latter gradually become longer and eventually the clonic movements cease altogether, marking the end of the seizure. Incontinence commonly occurs at the end of the clonic phase. The convulsion usually ceases after a few minutes and is followed by a post-ictal period of drowsiness, confusion, headache and sleep. It is not uncommon for people to fall deeply asleep after a convulsion and this may sometimes be misinterpreted as unconsciousness. When they wake up they will be unaware of what has

Convulsive seizures are common

Deep sleep after a convulsion

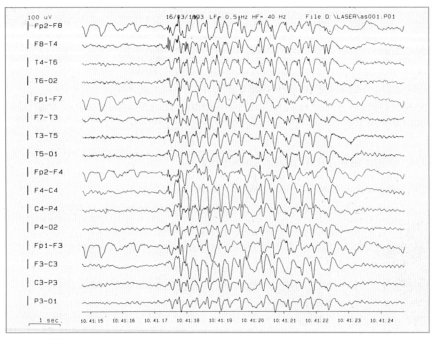

Figure 3. EEG showing 3 per second spike and wave discharges in primary generalized epilepsy. (Courtesy of Dr Li Li Min).

happened, will often feel lethargic, and may complain of generalized muscle aches due to the strenuous muscle activity of the clonic phase.

ABSENCE SEIZURES

Typical absence attacks, previously known as "petit mal", are a much rarer form of generalized seizure. *They occur almost exclusively in childhood and early adolescence.* The child suddenly appears blank and stares: fluttering of the eyelids, swallowing, and flopping of the head may occur. The attacks last only a few seconds and often pass unrecognized. Not infrequently, they are diagnosed only when learning difficulties at school are investigated in a child who has problems concentrating due to frequent absence attacks. Absence attacks are associated with a characteristic EEG pattern, the so-called 3 per second generalized spike-and-wave discharges (Figure 3). They may be precipitated by hyperventilation, which is a useful diagnostic maneuver.

MYOCLONIC SEIZURES

Myoclonic seizures are abrupt, very brief, involuntary flexion movements which may involve the whole body, or part of it, for example the arms or head. They occur most commonly in the morning, shortly after waking. They may sometimes cause the patient to fall, but recovery is immediate. The majority of myoclonic seizures occur in relatively benign seizure conditions but sometimes they herald more severe disorders. Not all myoclonus is the result of epilepsy: non-epileptic myoclonic jerks occur in a variety of other neurological conditions including lesions of the brainstem and spinal cord. Myoclonus is usually termed "epileptic" if it occurs in the context of a seizure disorder without evidence of encephalopathy, at least initially, and "symptomatic" if it accompanies an encephalopathy, which is the predominant feature. Examples of conditions often accompanied by myoclonus are acute cerebral hypoxia or ischemia, and degenerative brain diseases such at Creutzfeld-Jakob disease. In addition, *myoclonic seizures may also occur in healthy people*, particularly when they are just going off to sleep (hypnic jerk, hypnogogic myoclonus or nocturnal start), and are then considered to be a normal physiological phenomenon.

Abrupt, brief, involuntary flexion movements

May occur in healthy people

ATONIC AND TONIC SEIZURES

These types of generalized attacks are very rare, accounting for less than 1% of the epileptic attacks seen in the general population. They usually occur during the course of some forms of severe epilepsy, often starting in early childhood, such as the Lennox-Gastaut syndrome or myoclonic astatic epilepsy. Atonic seizures (sometimes called akinetic attacks or drop attacks) involve a sudden loss of tone in the postural muscles, and the patient falls to the ground. There are no convulsive movements. Recovery is rapid, with no perceptible post-ictal symptomatology. During tonic seizures, there is a sudden increase in the muscle tone of the body and the patient becomes rigid, usually falling backwards onto the ground. Again, recovery is generally rapid. *Tonic and atonic attacks are often accompanied by severe injury.*

Less than 1% of epileptic attacks

2.5 How are the epileptic syndromes classified?

In addition to classifying epileptic seizures by type, a number of distinctive epileptic syndromes have been recognized (a syndrome being a specific constellation of symptoms and signs). In the case of epilepsy, the features of the seizures, the presence of characteristic structural lesions, age of onset, positive family history, and typical changes in the EEG usually define syndromes. It is important to try to categorize epilepsies according to the syndromic classification if possible, since this may have implications both for prognosis and treatment; in addition, it may prove possible to anticipate particular complications of certain syndromes. However, not all patients with chronic seizure disorders fit into such a classification.

Distinctive epileptic syndromes

A classification scheme for epileptic syndromes and related disorders proposed by the ILAE, although controversial and with a number of limitations, *is used in most tertiary referral centers*[3] (Table 2). A new five-axis classification scheme has recently being proposed by ILAE but has not yet been widely adopted. The scheme mostly in use classifies epileptic syndromes into four groups: localization-related (partial or focal), generalized, undetermined and special syndromes. Within these groups the syndromes are further divided into three sub-groups: primary or idiopathic, secondary or symptomatic, and cryptogenic. When epileptic seizures are the only symptom of an inherited or genetic disorder, the syndrome is termed primary or idiopathic; when they occur as symptoms of a condition associated with structural brain lesions, the syndrome is termed symptomatic or secondary, and when the etiology of the condition is unknown the term cryptogenic is used. The terms "idiopathic" and "cryptogenic" are sometimes used interchangeably for disorders in which the specific etiology has not been identified. *This should, however, be avoided, and the term "idiopathic" reserved for those syndromes which are presumed to be inherited.*

Classification scheme

"Idiopathic" refers to an inherited disorder

Epileptic seizures always indicate an abnormal process, but not all seizures are indicative of a chronic seizure disorder. Under the right circumstances (for example, following a head injury or in the context of acute hypoglycemia), it may be possible to trigger a seizure in any individual. Acute symptomatic seizures or situation-related seizures,

Indication of an abnormal process

1. **LOCALIZATION-RELATED** (FOCAL, LOCAL, PARTIAL)

    1.1 Idiopathic (primary)

        Benign childhood epilepsy with centro-temporal spikes
        Childhood epilepsy with occipital paroxysms
        Primary reading epilepsy

    1.2 Symptomatic (secondary)

        Temporal lobe epilepsies
        Frontal lobe epilepsies
        Parietal lobe epilepsies
        Occipital lobe epilepsies
        Chronic progressive epilepsia partialis continua of childhood
        Syndromes characterized by seizures with specific modes of precipitation

    1.3 Cryptogenic

        Defined by:

        Seizure type
        Clinical features
        Etiology
        Anatomical localization

2. **GENERALIZED**

    2.1 Idiopathic (with age-related onset – listed in order of age)

        Benign neonatal familial convulsions
        Benign neonatal convulsions
        Benign myoclonic epilepsy in infancy
        Childhood absence epilepsy
        Juvenile absence epilepsy
        Juvenile myoclonic epilepsy
        Epilepsies with grand mal seizures on awakening
        Other generalized idiopathic epilepsies
        Epilepsies with seizures precipitated by specific modes of activation.

    2.2 Cryptogenic or symptomatic

        West syndrome
        Lennox-Gastaut syndrome
        Epilepsy with myoclonic-astatic seizures
        Epilepsy with myoclonic absences

    2.3 Symptomatic

        2.3.1 Non-specific etiology

            Early myoclonic encephalopathy
            Early infantile epileptic encephalopathy with suppression bursts
            Other symptomatic generalized epilepsies

2.3.2 Specific syndromes

Epileptic seizures may complicate many disease states

3. **EPILEPSIES AND SYNDROMES**
(UNDETERMINED WHETHER FOCAL OR GENERALIZED)

3.1 With both generalized and focal seizures

Neonatal seizures
Severe myoclonic epilepsy in infancy
Electrical status epilepticus during slow wave sleep – rare condition
Acquired epileptic aphasia
Other undetermined epilepsies

3.2 Without unequivocal generalized or focal features

4. **SPECIAL SYNDROMES**

4.1 Situation-related seizures

Febrile convulsions
Isolated seizures or isolated status epilepticus
Seizures occurring only when there is an acute or toxic event due to factors such as alcohol, drugs, eclampsia, nonketotic hyperglycemia

Epilepsia 1989, 30:389-399

Table 2. *International Classification of Epilepsies, Epileptic Syndromes and related disorders.*

which occur as a result of chemical or physiological insult to the brain, although listed in the ILAE classification of epileptic syndromes (under special syndromes), are not generally considered epileptic disorders in their own right.

2.6 What are the characteristics of the main epileptic syndromes?

Many of the epileptic syndromes start in childhood or adolescence, and are therefore sometimes called age-linked epilepsies. The more common epileptic syndromes are discussed below:

Age-linked epilepsies

1.0 Localization-related epileptic syndromes

1.1 Idiopathic localization-related syndromes

Rolandic epilepsy, also known as benign partial epilepsy of childhood or benign epilepsy of childhood with centrotemporal spikes, *is the most common syndrome in this group of seizure disorders.* The onset of seizures is between the ages of two and 14 years, usually between 5 and 10 years. This syndrome may account for up to 15% of epilepsy in this age group. Children with benign partial epilepsy of childhood usually have simple partial seizures, occasionally with progression to complex partial or secondarily generalized seizures. Seizures tend to occur during the night or on awakening in the morning, and usually involve the face, lips and the tongue. The interictal EEG tracing has a characteristic appearance in this syndrome: it consists of frequent paroxysms of slow spike and wave discharges over the centrotemporal ("rolandic") region, with a normal background rhythm. About 30% of the children have a family history of epilepsy. There are no neurological or intellectual abnormalities associated with this condition and it has an excellent prognosis for complete seizure remission by the time of puberty. Long-term treatment is usually not required.

> Rolandic epilepsy

Benign occipital epilepsy is a syndrome with a number of similarities to benign rolandic epilepsy, but the EEG disturbance is in the occipital lobe and the children may present with nausea and visual disturbances during the seizures.

> Benign occipital epilepsy

1.2   Symptomatic localization-related epilepsies and

1.3   Cryptogenic localization-related epilepsies

Syndromes in these groups are defined by the clinical manifestations of the seizures and by the lobe of the brain in which they originate, regardless of the background etiology. Possible etiological factors include mesial temporal sclerosis (Ammon's horn), indolent gliomas, cortical dysplasias, cerebral infarction, hamartomas, angiomas, tuberous sclerosis, glial scars and meningiomas. In about a third of cases no etiology is found but it is likely that with improvements in imaging techniques, the cryptogenic cases will become progressively less common.

> Clinical manifestations

TEMPORAL LOBE SEIZURES

Approximately 60-70% of localization-related epilepsies originate in the temporal lobes. Simple partial, complex partial and secondarily generalized seizures with a large variety of

> Originate in the temporal lobes

clinical manifestations may occur as a result of temporal lobe abnormalities. Because of this diversity they are often very difficult to classify. The majority of seizures of temporal lobe origin begin in the hippocampus or amygdala. Autonomic symptoms, impaired consciousness and automatisms are the principal manifestations of these seizures. Loss of awareness suggests the involvement of both temporal lobes, and may or may not be preceded by a simple partial seizure (an aura).

A strange "rising" sensation in the epigastrium, and anomalies of smell or taste, often of an offensive nature, are common. Patients may undergo autonomic changes, becoming pale or flushed, and with pupillary dilatation, sweating and changes in heart rate. Patients having temporal lobe seizures may experience various psychic phenomena. These include dysmnestic symptoms (for example, déjà vu, jamais vu) and affective experiences (such as exhilaration, fear or anger). Patients may also have auditory or visual hallucinations or illusions. Spontaneous or reactive automatisms may occur, of which oroalimentary (lip-smacking, chewing, swallowing) and motor (drinking, undressing, fumbling, rubbing and walking) automatisms are the most common. Vocalization ranging from grunts to repeated words and sentences may also occur. These symptoms may be present in isolation as a simple partial seizure, or in a variety of combinations as complex partial seizures. Both may progress to secondarily generalized seizures.

FRONTAL LOBE SEIZURES

About 20-30% of localization-related epilepsies originate in the frontal lobes. Simple partial, complex partial and secondarily generalized seizures may occur as a result of frontal lobe discharges. Some frontal lobe seizures, particularly those arising from the motor areas, are easy to classify, while others, particularly those originating from the prefrontal, cingulate and orbitofrontal areas can easily be confused with temporal lobe seizures. Frontal lobe seizures are usually of short duration, often starting and stopping abruptly, and not infrequently occur in clusters.

Adversive attacks, with deviation of head and eyes to one side at the onset of the attack, *are common manifestations of frontal lobe seizures.* They are often associated with clonic movements of a limb on that side or with limb posturing. Motor automatisms and autonomic symptoms may also occur. Speech arrest may be

Common manifestations of frontal lobe seizures

present, particularly if the seizure originates in the dominant hemisphere, while vocalization may indicate a non-dominant seizure. Atonic seizures, sometimes causing severe injury, may occur when there is a rapid spread of discharges from one hemisphere to the other. On occasion these evolve into generalized tonic clonic seizures, usually with a rapid recovery afterwards. Post-ictal phenomena such as dysphasia and hemiparesis not infrequently follow seizures of frontal lobe origin: the nature of such phenomena may provide a clue to the location of the epileptic focus.

PARIETAL AND OCCIPITAL LOBE SEIZURES

About 10% of all localization-related epilepsies originate in the parietal and occipital lobes. Those originating in the parietal lobe often have rather non-specific features, so that the site of origin is not immediately obvious, although somatosensory disturbances may feature in the symptomatology. *Seizures originating in the occipital lobes are characterized by visual phenomena.* These seizures usually present as simple partial seizures but often spread anteriorly leading to complex partial seizures with predominantly frontal or temporal lobe phenomenology. Secondarily generalized convulsions may also occur.

Characterized by visual phenomena

Somatosensory experiences of parietal origin include localized sensations (tingling, prickling, numbness, crawling or shock-like sensations), pain and changes in temperature. On rare occasions, parietal seizures may manifest themselves as abnormalities of body image, such as a feeling of movement in an immobile limb, a sensation of floating of a body part, or the feeling of absence of a body part. Apraxia, acalculia, alexia, sexual phenomenology and vertiginous sensations may also occasionally occur in parietal lobe epilepsy.

Elementary visual hallucinations, especially crude sensations of light and color, *are the most common manifestations of occipital epilepsy.* These hallucinations may consist of various patterns, usually moving out of the visual field. Transient amaurosis as part of a seizure or as a post-ictal phenomenon may also occur. In young children occipital seizures may take the form of nocturnal bouts of vomiting associated with tonic deviation of the eyes, sometimes with secondary generalization.

Visual hallucinations – manifestations of occipital epilepsy

EPILEPSIA PARTIALIS CONTINUA

This is a rare form of severe chronic epilepsy, which in the majority of patients starts in the first decade of life. Patients present with simple partial seizures that become almost continuous: progression to complex partial seizures and secondarily generalized seizures may occur. In some patients, the development of epilepsia partialis continua heralds the onset of a rare condition called Rasmussen's encephalitis (chronic encephalitis and epilepsy). This is an unusual syndrome usually occurring in childhood, and characterized by the development of intractable partial seizures, progressive hemiparesis and intellectual deterioration. Pathologically, changes of chronic encephalitis are seen, almost invariably affecting one cerebral hemisphere only. The etiology is unclear, although there may be an autoimmune mechanism. The condition sometimes seems to stabilize after a period of years, but not before considerable neurological damage has occurred. Other lesions which may cause epilepsia partialis continua at any age include cortical dysplasia, neoplasia or vascular malformations. Antiepileptic therapy is often ineffective and surgical treatment may be necessary.

Rare form of severe chronic epilepsy

2.0   Generalized epilepsies and syndromes

2.1   Idiopathic generalized epilepsy or primary generalized epilepsy

The most common of the epileptic syndromes are the idiopathic generalized epilepsies or the primary generalized epilepsies (2.1 in Table 2). The syndromes contained in this group account for about one third of all epilepsies *and have a typical EEG pattern with paroxysms of generalized "3 per second spike and wave" discharges* (Figure 3) which may be induced by overbreathing and photic stimulation (photosensitivity). Patients often have a family history of generalized epilepsy, suggesting that genetic factors are important. The onset of seizures in this group is usually between the ages of five and 15 years, although occasionally they develop in younger children. There is no sex bias and *either sex may be affected*.

Primary generalized epilepsies

The seizure types seen in these syndromes are generalized tonic clonic seizures, typical absence seizures and myoclonic seizures, on their own or in different combinations. Within these syndromes, generalized tonic clonic seizures are usually seen much less frequently than myoclonic or absence seizures. *There is a tendency for both generalized tonic clonic convulsions and myoclonic seizures to occur early in the morning,* either on awakening or within half-an-hour of waking. The majority of patients in this group find that seizures (of any type) may be triggered by sleep deprivation, and in some, photosensitivity is also a feature. Patients who are photosensitive may have seizures in association with flickering lights caused by natural phenomena such as the reflection of the sun on water, travelling in a car along a tree-lined boulevard with the sun in the background, or by artificial causes such as flickering lights in a discotheque, television screens or electronic games. Occasionally a patient's first seizure happens to occur in the context of such a precipitant, which may then be blamed for the development of epilepsy, although underlying photosensitivity can often be demonstrated. It should be stressed, however, that **the majority of people with epilepsy are not photosensitive,** and discotheques, computer games and so on should not adversely affect them.

> Tendency for early morning occurrences

Benign neonatal familial convulsions, benign myoclonic epilepsy in infancy and childhood, juvenile typical absence-type epilepsy, juvenile myoclonic epilepsy and epilepsy with generalized tonic clonic convulsions on awakening are all types of generalized idiopathic epilepsy. *The prognosis for full seizure control and long-term remission in all these forms is usually very good as treatment with specific antiepileptic drugs is highly effective.* Most patients may expect to be able to tail off antiepileptic medication after a number of years in remission. However, in the case of some syndromes, particularly *juvenile myoclonic epilepsy, there is a high relapse rate on discontinuation of medication.*

> Treatment with antiepileptic medication is highly effective

2.2 and 2.3 Generalized symptomatic or cryptogenic epilepsies

Generalized symptomatic or cryptogenic epilepsies include **the so-called West syndrome and the Lennox-Gastaut syndrome,** which **have some features in common.** Both occur more commonly in males, and have their onset in childhood. In approximately 30% of cases the child is normal until the seizures start, but development then becomes impaired, sometimes progressively. In the remaining cases, the epileptic condition is preceded by neurological abnormalities or developmental delay. It is believed that a common physiopathologic mechanism is responsible for both conditions, the differences in presentation occurring as a result of the differing degree of brain maturation.

> West syndrome and the Lennox-Gastaut syndrome

An English physician originally described West syndrome in 1841 in his own baby son. *The terms infantile spasms, salaam spasms and hypsarrhythmia have also been used to refer to this syndrome.* The onset is usually around the age of six months (range three-nine months), and the child may have identifiable brain damage (such as tuberous sclerosis, cortical dysplasia, malformations, or anoxic-ischemic insults) prior to the onset, but in about one-third of cases no etiology can be found. In this syndrome a characteristic EEG pattern, termed hypsarrhythmia, is seen. This consists of a chaotic pattern of high amplitude irregular slow activity intermixed with multifocal spike and sharp wave discharges. The seizures may be flexor, extensor, or mixed, the latter type being most common. Flexor spasms consist of sudden flexion of the neck, arms and legs. Sudden flexion of the trunk produces so-called "salaam" or "jack-knife" seizures. During extensor spasms, sudden movement of the neck, trunk and legs occurs, while in mixed spasms, there is flexion of the neck, trunk and arm, and extension of the legs. Seizures often occur in clusters, particularly soon after the child has been awoken. *The prognosis for West syndrome is guarded.* Overall, only about 20% of children make a complete recovery, with death at a young age occurring in a further 20%. Almost two-thirds of survivors have ongoing epilepsy, and up to 50% have persistent neurological handicap. The response to treatment with conventional antiepileptic drugs is poor in West syndrome, but in some children the outcome may be improved if vigabatrin is given early in the condition. This drug appears particularly helpful in children in whom the condition is associated with tuberous sclerosis. Adrenocorticotrophic hormone (ACTH) and nitrazepam may also be helpful in the management of infantile spasms.

Infantile spasms

The Lennox-Gastaut syndrome is characterized by multiple seizure types including tonic and atonic seizures and complex absences. Tonic-clonic convulsions and myoclonic seizures may occur. It is a rare condition, accounting for perhaps 1% of all new cases of epilepsy, although due to its poor outcome it may represent as many as 10% of cases of severe epilepsy. *Lennox-Gastaut syndrome is frequently associated with learning difficulties and other co-morbidities.* In about half of the cases no definite etiological factor can be identified, although it is recognized that some of these are symptomatic rather than truly "cryptogenic". A past history of West syndrome is the most common identifiable cause, being present in 30-40% of children. Other causes include brain damage at birth, infections, tumor and severe head trauma. The condition

Multiple seizure types

Associated with learning difficulties

typically has its onset between the ages of three and five years, though it may start as early as one year or as late as 8 years of age (rarely even older). Patients are at high risk of developing status epilepticus, which may be either tonic-clonic or non-convulsive. *The prognosis of Lennox-Gastaut is very poor,* both with regard to seizure control (seizures persisting in 60-80% of patients) and mental development. Cognitive and behavioral problems are very common, and it is unusual for patients ever to lead independent lives.

Poor prognosis

The EEG pattern in Lennox-Gastaut syndrome is almost invariably abnormal even interictally (Figure 4). The background activity is slow, and 2-2.5Hz spike and wave and polyspike and wave discharges, often most marked over the anterior and posterior head regions, are characteristically seen. Such discharges may sometimes dominate the EEG for hours or days at a time. The complexes are not usually induced by hyperventilation or by photic stimulation. Rhythmic 10Hz spikes are seen particularly during slow-wave sleep.

The syndrome of epilepsy with myoclonic-astatic seizures has many similarities to the Lennox-Gastaut syndrome, but can be differentiated by the prominence of myoclonic seizures, the fact that the majority of people have a previously normal neurological history, and by the absence of the characteristic EEG

Myoclonic-astatic seizures

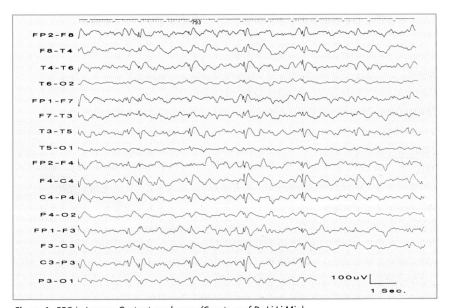

Figure 4. EEG in Lennox-Gastaut syndrome. (Courtesy of Dr Li Li Min).

pattern. Tonic seizures, characteristic of Lennox-Gastaut syndrome, only occur late in patients in whom the condition is severe. In one-third of cases there is a family history. The prognosis for mental development and seizure control is rather variable: seizure frequency may provide some indication of the probable overall outcome.

3.0   Epilepsies and syndromes undetermined whether focal or generalized

NEONATAL SEIZURES

Neonatal seizures occur in the first four weeks of life, in about 0.5% of babies. The syndrome is defined solely by age of onset, with no regard for the background etiology or ictal manifestations. Causes of neonatal seizures include infection, anoxia, ischemia, trauma, metabolic imbalance and nutritional disturbances. In about one-quarter of cases no etiological factor is identified. In a few babies the seizures occur on a genetic basis. Seizures are often subtle and include clonic movements, eye deviation and blinking, usually of short duration: very rarely, more conventional seizure types may occur. *The clinical features of the seizures probably reflect the immaturity of the neonatal brain.*

First four weeks of life

Immaturity of the neonatal brain

The EEG in the neonate is often difficult to interpret, but it may be possible to identify an epileptic focus. The prognosis is related to the underlying pathology, but the overall outcome is not good; approximately 25% die in the first year of life, and about half either carry on having seizures into adult life or have evidence of neurological damage, such as learning disability or cerebral palsy.

25% make a full recovery

Only about 25% make a full recovery. Indicators of poor prognosis include prematurity, early onset of seizures (especially in the first two days of life), focal cerebral lesions or malformations, intracranial bleeding and the presence of a very abnormal EEG. However, some syndromes of "benign" neonatal convulsions have been recognized. These include benign idiopathic neonatal convulsions ("fifth day fits"), which are said to account for about 5% of neonatal seizures, although some studies have suggested that they may represent one-third of all neonatal seizures. Benign familial neonatal convulsions have an autosomal dominant inheritance, the gene being mapped to the long arm of chromosome 20.

SEVERE MYOCLONIC EPILEPSY IN INFANCY

This is a rare condition that affects infants in the first year of life. It presents with generalized clonic convulsions and myoclonic seizures. The EEG shows generalized spike and wave discharges and marked photosensitivity. Most cases have recently been associated with a mutation in an ion channel gene. Antiepileptic treatment is not effective and the prognosis for seizure control, mental and motor development is poor. Recently, however, it has being reported that some patients with this condition may respond to stiripentol, a new antiepileptic drug which has an orphan drug indication for this condition.

ACQUIRED EPILEPTIC APHASIA

This condition, also known as **Landau-Kleffner syndrome, is a rare disorder** in which persisting aphasia develops in association with severe focal EEG abnormalities. It occurs more commonly in boys than girls and has its onset in childhood, usually

Landau-Kleffner syndrome is a rare disorder

between the ages of four and seven years. The condition usually occurs in children with previously normal development and the etiology is unknown. The first sign is usually a progressive acquired aphasia, commonly followed by generalized and partial epileptic seizures, although in about 30% of patients no clinical seizures are noted, while in some children seizures may precede the onset of the language disturbance. Motor speech function is affected, often leading to an almost total mutism. Behavioral disturbances are observed in the majority of patients. The EEG recording shows a multi-focal spike and wave pattern, the epileptic activity most often being seen in the temporal and parieto-occipital regions.

Favorable prognosis

The prognosis for seizure control is usually favorable, but the outcome of the language disturbance is guarded. In some patients speech may be regained by adulthood, but there may be severe psychosocial consequences as a result of the prolonged aphasia.

EPILEPSY WITH CONTINUOUS SPIKE-WAVES DURING SLOW WAVE SLEEP

This condition, also known as electrical status epilepticus during slow wave sleep (ESES) **is another rare form of childhood epilepsy** which has as its hallmark an EEG pattern consisting of almost continuous slow spike and wave discharges during most of non-REM sleep. The condition usually starts during the first decade

Electrical status epilepticus – rare condition

of life and the child may present with several different seizure types, both diurnal and nocturnal, including focal motor, complex partial, tonic clonic, absence and atonic seizures. The etiology is unknown, although about 20-30% of cases are associated with identifiable brain pathology (for example, previous meningitis, birth asphyxia, cytomegalovirus infection). In most patients there is an arrest of mental development at the time of onset, and severe behavioral disturbances may develop. *The prognosis for seizure control is good*, and the electrical status epilepticus generally remits around puberty, although learning difficulties and behavioral disorders usually persist.

4.0   Special syndromes

4.1   Situation-related seizures

Acute head trauma, fever, sleep deprivation, use of convulsant drugs, withdrawal of sedative drugs or alcohol, reversible central nervous system infections, eclampsia, metabolic imbalance, and toxic states can cause epileptic seizures, either single or recurrent, in susceptible individuals, without constituting an epileptic disorder. These seizures are called acute symptomatic seizures or situation-related seizures. They usually take the form of generalized tonic clonic convulsions. Long-term treatment is not usually required, except in instances in which the seizures recur after the triggering factor has been removed or corrected.

FEBRILE CONVULSIONS

Febrile seizures occur in the context of a febrile illness, often of viral etiology, in children between the ages of six months and six years. They affect as many as 3% of children in the general population and there is often a family history of febrile convulsions or epilepsy. The seizures usually take the form of short generalized tonic clonic convulsions, without other features, in toddlers with body temperatures over 38°C, and occur particularly following a rapid rise in temperature. Acute treatment, in addition to supportive management, consists of diazepam, either rectally or intravenously, reducing the child's temperature by means of sponging, cooling with a fan, and paracetamol if necessary, and treatment of the underlying condition if appropriate. Febrile convulsions do not usually require long-term prophylactic treatment unless complications develop. However, parents should be counseled about the risk of recurrences

Occur in febrile illness

and measures to avoid these. Risks for recurrence include age less than 15 months, epilepsy or febrile convulsions in first-degree relatives, and prolonged first febrile seizure. In some children intermittent prophylaxis with a benzodiazepine is helpful. EEG is usually not indicated.

The most important differential diagnosis in this condition is with seizures that are triggered by central nervous system infections such as meningitis, encephalitis and brain abscess. If there is any doubt about the diagnosis, a lumbar puncture is indicated, provided there are no features to suggest raised intracranial pressure. If there is a suspicion of this, the child should be transferred to a specialist center with neurosurgical facilities for CT scan before lumbar puncture is performed. In this instance, the need for appropriate antibiotic treatment prior to transfer should be considered.

Importance of differential diagnosis

In the great majority of children presenting with febrile convulsions, even if recurrent, the overall prognosis is excellent with no further seizures or other problems. However, in a few children, chronic seizures subsequently develop, so that the risk of epilepsy by the age of 25 years is about 7%. The risk is greatest in children with prolonged convulsions (lasting more than 20-30 minutes), those with previous signs of developmental delay, and those with partial seizures. The probability of epilepsy subsequently developing is also greater in children with a family history of afebrile seizures in a first degree relative.

Excellent prognosis

2.7 What factors may precipitate seizures in people with epilepsy?

In the majority of patients with epileptic seizures, seizures happen in a random fashion and are totally unpredictable. However, some patients are able to identify certain conditions which may trigger their seizures. If such factors exist and can be identified, measures can be taken to avoid them, thus reducing the likelihood of further attacks. Examples of *factors that may trigger seizures in some patients are flickering lights, sleep deprivation, stressful situations, fear and anger.* Other people are liable to have seizures when they take certain drugs or alcohol.

Random and totally unpredictable

Factors which may trigger seizures

Women with epilepsy often complain that their seizures are more frequent around the time of their menstrual period, probably as a result of hormonal changes and fluid retention. A few of these women are helped by additional medication in the week prior to and during menstruation.

2.8   What are nocturnal seizures?

A proportion of people with seizures have most or even all of their attacks during the night. This type of epilepsy may prove difficult to diagnose since seizures are often not witnessed. *If there is a suspicion of nocturnal seizures, it is important that investigations are carried out since the majority of these patients have seizures of partial origin, and there may be an underlying structural lesion.* There may also be implications for treatment, and many patients with nocturnal seizures without a progressive cause elect not to take antiepileptic drugs. However, the risk of sudden unexpected death in epilepsy (SUDEP) needs to be considered when taking such a decision.

Seizures of partial origin may have an underlying structural lesion

2.9   What is status epilepticus?

The great majority of seizures are self-limiting, that is, they stop spontaneously. On occasion, however, *seizures occur in quick succession, without any period of recovery between one attack and the next, a situation known as status epilepticus.* This may occur with any type of seizure, but is particularly dangerous if it involves generalized tonic clonic convulsions, when it constitutes a medical emergency.

2.10   What are the features of tonic clonic status epilepticus?

Tonic clonic status epilepticus occurs when a tonic clonic seizure (or recurrent tonic clonic seizures without recovery in between) continues for at least 30 minutes. The EEG during this period shows almost continuous ictal activity. The annual incidence of tonic clonic status epilepticus has been estimated to be about 20 - 30 cases per 100,000 people. About half of cases occur in people with established epilepsy; in the remainder, it occurs as an initial or isolated epileptic phenomenon. *About 5% of all people with epilepsy have at least one episode of tonic clonic status epilepticus in their life.* It is more common in children, in people with learning difficulties and in those with structural cerebral pathology, particularly if this involves the frontal lobes.

Tonic clonic seizures continue for at least 30 minutes

In patients with established epilepsy a precipitating factor can be identified in over 50% of cases. *The most important is acute antiepileptic drug withdrawal, either due to poor compliance or under medical supervision.* Other precipitants include withdrawal of other drugs or alcohol, infections, other intercurrent illness or progression of the underlying lesion. In patients presenting with tonic clonic status epilepticus as the first sign of epilepsy, an expanding intracerebral lesion must be ruled out. Other causes of tonic clonic status epilepticus as an initial epileptic phenomenon include head trauma, cerebrovascular disease, and encephalitis.

A common problem in the management of people with tonic clonic status is that of misdiagnosis. It is our experience that the majority of people referred to tertiary referral centers from other hospitals in presumed status epilepticus do not have the condition. Pseudostatus epilepticus is the most common diagnosis in these patients, and such patients may be identified by EEG monitoring.

The problem of misdiagnosis

Tonic clonic status epilepticus carries a high mortality and neurological morbidity. About 10% of patients with tonic clonic status epilepticus die, usually of the underlying condition. Permanent neurological damage and mental deterioration may result from status, particularly in young children. The longer the duration of the status epilepticus, the more the risk of neurological morbidity is increased.

2.11 What are the manifestations of non-convulsive status epilepticus?

Non-convulsive status epilepticus occurs when prolonged or recurrent minor seizures or subclinical ictal activity persist for 30 minutes or more. Although any non-convulsive seizure type may cause this form of status the most common presentations are absence status, atypical absence status and complex partial status. They do not constitute a medical emergency in the same manner as tonic clonic status epilepticus, but it has been argued that prolonged temporal lobe seizure activity may contribute to subsequent memory difficulties. Benzodiazepines are often helpful in treatment, although many cases resolve spontaneously, sometimes with the development of a tonic clonic seizure.

Subclinical ictal activity persists for 30 minutes

2.12 What is absence status?

Absence status occurs in up to 5% of patients with childhood typical absence-type epilepsy. The hallmark of absence status is clouding of consciousness and behavioral change, which may be present in various degrees of severity. Confusion and disorientation sometimes occur. The eyes may be partially closed, and the patient appears in a trance-like state. *The EEG is diagnostic, showing continuous or almost continuous bilaterally synchronous spike and wave activity, with little or no reactivity to sensory stimuli.* Precipitating features can be identified in a minority of cases, and include withdrawal of medication, hypoglycemia, hyperventilation, flashing or bright lights, sleep deprivation, fatigue or stress. Most patients have known typical absence epilepsy but occasionally absence status is the first manifestation of epilepsy. Patients may suffer repeated attacks, which in the majority of instances last 12 hours or less, although they may persist for days or weeks. A highly characteristic feature of absence status is the termination of the episode by a generalized tonic clonic seizure. Amnesia is usual for the episode but variable though short patches of recall may punctuate it. The occurrence of episodes of absence status does not seem to prejudice the overall good prognosis of childhood typical absence-type epilepsy.

> Continuous bilaterally synchronous spikes

2.13 What are the features of atypical absence status?

Atypical absence status is common among patients with the Lennox-Gastaut syndrome. It takes the form of a fluctuating confusional or stuporose state with frequent myoclonic seizures. It is often preceded by alterations in the general physical and psychological state, with changes in the patient's motor activity, mood or intellectual attainment, sometimes lasting for hours or days before the overt status develops, and raising the possibility of subclinical non-convulsive status. The status may evolve gradually, and tonic status may eventually develop. Diffuse slow spike and wave dominates the EEG but is often similar to the usual interictal pattern seen in this condition. The usual therapies for status are generally ineffective. The occurrence of atypical absence status in the Lennox-Gastaut syndrome does not seem to be related to outcome.

2.14 How does complex partial status epilepticus present?

Complex partial status epilepticus was until recently considered to be a rare form of epilepsy but it is now recognized that episodes of status complicate the course of many partial epilepsies: *they are more common than other types of non-convulsive status or tonic clonic status.* The clinical features are variable, but the manifestations are not simply prolonged or reiterated versions of isolated complex partial seizures. *The cardinal features of complex partial status are confusion and altered consciousness, which may fluctuate or be almost continuous.* The features that may be encountered vary from profound stupor with little response to external stimuli in some patients, to a state in which no discernible confusion is present, but cognitive testing reveals subtle abnormalities. Alterations in posture, convulsive movements, and tonic spasms may all occur intermittently in complex partial status. Adversion of the head and eyes is common. Motor features, including adversion, are more common in frontal status than in temporal complex partial status. Myoclonic jerks, posturing, and orofacial and other motor automatisms also occur. Behavioral changes range from agitation to severe psychomotor retardation and stupor, but in some patients, behavior may be almost normal. Speech patterns may be markedly altered, with perseveration, confabulation, echolalia, repetitive utterances or stereotyped responses. Patients in a state of complex partial status characteristically say very little, and responses to questions, although eventually appropriate, may show a marked delay between question and answer.

In some patients, psychotic features are prominent, with delusions, hallucinations, illogical responses, and often a curious perseverative obsession with opposites, such as black/white, good/bad, left/right. Prolonged dreamy states with altered perception of time or space may occur. *A psychiatric misdiagnosis is common where psychotic features are prominent,* and some patients have histories of psychiatric hospital admissions before the epileptic nature of the event is recognized.

Psychotic features are prominent

Psychiatric misdiagnosis is common

The patient usually has amnesia for the whole episode. Patients with extratemporal status are said to have less alteration of consciousness and amnesia than those with status arising in the temporal lobe. Complex partial status has no characteristic or consistent scalp EEG pattern. Although seldom normal, the interictal and ictal recordings in complex partial status may be very similar, and a whole range of EEG patterns may be seen. Several different ictal patterns may be demonstrable, including continuous or frequent spike or spike and slow wave discharges, which may be widespread or local.

CHAPTER 3

THE EPIDEMIOLOGY OF EPILEPSY

3.1 What are the difficulties of studying the epidemiology of epilepsy?

The epidemiology of epilepsy refers to the characteristics and dynamics of epilepsy in the community. *There are immense difficulties in establishing precise epidemiological statistics for a heterogeneous condition like epilepsy.* Unlike most ailments, epilepsy is episodic. Between seizures, both the clinical examination and laboratory investigations of patients may be perfectly normal. The diagnosis is, therefore, essentially a clinical one, relying on the patient's account of his seizures, and, often more importantly, on the description given by an eyewitness. The difficulties of diagnosis are compounded by the fact that there is a variety of other conditions in which consciousness may be transiently impaired, which may be confused with epilepsy.

Difficult to establish precise epidemiological statistics

Another problem in determining the epidemiology of epilepsy lies in the area of case identification[1]. Sometimes patients may be unaware of the nature of their attacks and hence not seek medical help. Patients with infrequent or mild seizures may not receive ongoing medical care and so may be missed in epidemiological surveys. Furthermore, since *in the past there has been a considerable degree of stigma attached to epilepsy,* which to a lesser extent still exists today, patients may be reluctant to admit their condition.

Considerable degree of stigma

There are few data regarding the incidence and prevalence of specific epileptic syndromes, and most of the rates quoted below relate to the epilepsies in general.

3.2 What is the incidence of epilepsy?

Epilepsy is a very common condition. Its incidence (the number of new cases per given population per year) in developed countries has been estimated to be *between 40 and 60 cases per 100,000 persons*, while the cumulative incidence (the risk of having the condition at some time in one's life) is between 2 and 5%. In less privileged countries, the incidence may be in excess of 100 cases per 100,000 people.

Up to 100 cases per 100,000 persons

No consistent national or racial differences have been found, although it is thought that the incidence may be higher in the less wealthy segments of society.

The incidence is relatively high in the first two decades of life, but falls over the next few decades, only to increase again in later life, mainly as a result of seizures caused by cerebrovascular disease. The incidence of epilepsy according to age is shown in Figure 5.

3.3 What is the prevalence of epilepsy?

The prevalence of epilepsy is the number of cases in the population at a given time. It is important, in defining the prevalence of epilepsy, to distinguish between "active" and "inactive" epilepsy. Epilepsy is usually deemed to be

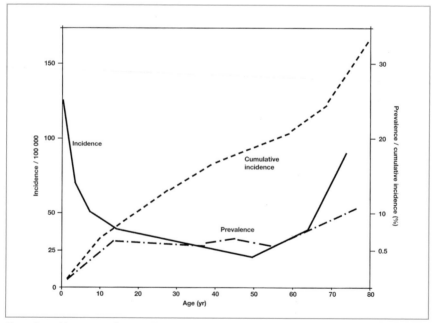

Figure 5. *Incidence, prevalence and cumulative incidence of epilepsy according to age. (Adapted from Hauser WA, Kurland LT. The epidemiology of epilepsy in Rochester, Minnesota, 1935 through 1967. Epilepsia 1975, 16:1-66).*

active if the patient has had at least one seizure in recent years (usually the past two years, although some investigators consider epilepsy to be active if patients have had seizures within the past five years), or if the patient continues to take antiepileptic medication. *Most studies of the prevalence of active epilepsy have estimated the figure to be between 4 and 10 per 1,000* (Figure 5). Cumulative incidence (lifetime prevalence) rates are much higher. It is estimated that between 2 and 5% of the population will have a non-febrile seizure at some point in time, and that seizures will recur in over 50%. Almost all reports show slightly higher rates in males than females.

Prevalence between 4 and 10 per 1,000 persons

Higher in males than females

3.4 What is the prognosis of epilepsy?

The prognosis for seizure control is quite good. As stated above, up to 5% of people will have at least one seizure in their lifetime. The prevalence of activity epilepsy is, however, much lower, suggesting that in most patients developing seizures, the condition eventually becomes inactive [2]. *Studies have shown that up to 70% of all people developing epilepsy will eventually become seizure-free and about half will successfully withdraw their medication.* Once a substantial period of remission has been achieved, the risk of further seizures is greatly reduced. A minority of patients (up to 30%) will develop chronic epilepsy, and in such cases, treatment is more difficult. Patients with symptomatic epilepsy, more than one seizure type, associated learning difficulties, or neurological or psychiatric disorders are more likely to develop a chronic seizure disorder. 5% of patients with intractable epilepsy will be unable to live in the community or will be dependent on others for their day-to-day needs, often because of associated handicaps. In a minority of patients with severe epilepsy, physical and intellectual deterioration may occur.

Up to 70% of all people with epilepsy will become seizure-free

3.5 What is the risk of recurrence after a first epileptic attack?

The orthodox viewpoint that single seizures should not be equated with epilepsy originates from the findings of early studies of recurrence, which suggested that a considerable proportion of patients with a single seizure had no further attacks. *Reported estimates of the risk of a second attack have varied from 27% by 3 years [3], to 84% after a variable period of follow up [4], depending on how the patient is identified after their first seizure and whether treatment is started after the initial event.*

Most studies in which patients have been identified very soon after their first attack (within one week or so) and not treated indicate that more than 50% of patients will have a recurrence [5,6]. It is well known that the risk of seizure recurrence is much higher in the first weeks or months after an initial attack. Consequently, if there is a long interval between the first seizure and registration into a recurrence study, a second seizure may have already occurred and the patient is therefore excluded from the study. From our own studies, the risk of recurrence also varies depending on the cause of the seizure (Figure 6) and the length of time for which patients remain seizure-free after their first attack (Figure 7).

3.6 What is the risk of recurrence of seizures after discontinuation of antiepileptic treatment?

60-70% of patients taking antiepileptic medication will eventually become seizure free. Because of the possible long-term side effects of the drugs, it is common clinical practice to consider drug withdrawal after a patient has had a substantial period of remission. Many studies have indicated a risk of relapse in doing so, the probability of this being of the order of 40% in adults and 20% in children after at least two years of freedom from seizures.

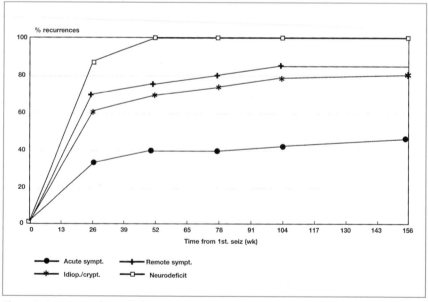

Figure 6. *Recurrence after a single seizure according to etiology (Adapted from Hart YM, Sander JW, Johnson AL, Shorvon SD. National General Practice Study of Epilepsy Recurrence after a first seizure. Lancet 1990, 336: 1271-1274).*

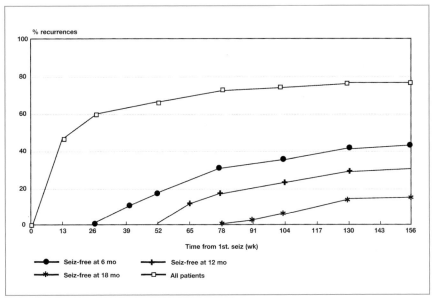

Figure 7. *Recurrence after a first seizure according to interval of seizure-freedom from initial event (Adapted from Hart YM, Sander JW, Johnson AL, Shorvon SD. National General Practice Study of Epilepsy Recurrence after a first seizure. Lancet 1990, 336: 1271-1274).*

Risk factors for recurrence include the presence of myoclonic seizures, structural abnormalities on brain scanning and long history of active epilepsy before the onset of remission.

3.7 What is the mortality of epilepsy?

Epilepsy is often assumed to be a benign condition with a low mortality. Although this is usually the case, *it does carry an increased mortality,* particularly in the case of younger patients and those with severe epilepsy [7].

Increased mortality in younger patients

3.8 Who is at risk of death from epilepsy?

It has consistently been reported that mortality rates are higher for males than females, although so far no convincing explanation has been advanced for this. The greatest increase in mortality rate is in those people aged less than 40 years, a group that has the smallest mortality in the general population. Conversely, the group in which epilepsy increases the risk of death least is among people aged 75 years or more, those people with the highest mortality rate from other causes.

The overall mortality rate has been estimated at two to three times greater than that of the general population, the increased risk being largely limited to the first 10 years after diagnosis. This suggests that the increased mortality is in part due to the underlying cause of epilepsy (brain tumors, head injury, vascular events, and so on), and this view is reinforced by the fact that even patients in whom seizures are completely controlled have an increased risk of death. Nonetheless, idiopathic generalized convulsions also confer an increased mortality.

Mortality rate greater than in the general population

Seizure type seems also to be relevant. The mortality of patients whose only seizure type is absence seizures is little different from that of the general population, while in patients with myoclonic seizures, mortality is increased four-fold. Higher mortality rates for non-whites of either sex, both for deaths due to and related to epilepsy, have been reported in the USA. This may, however, be related to socio-economic factors; infant mortality rates, a well-accepted measure of socio-economic deprivation, are almost twice as high among African Americans as in the white population.

Seizure type is relevant

3.9   What are the causes of death in epilepsy?

Common causes of death in people with epilepsy include chest infections, neoplasia and deaths directly related to seizures. Bronchopneumonia is an important cause of death in patients with epilepsy, particularly among the elderly although it is by no means confined to this age group. It seems likely that its occurrence in younger people is related to aspiration during a seizure, although this hypothesis has not been formally tested. Idiosyncratic side effects of some antiepileptic drugs have been associated with the death of patients, but are extremely rare events. Deaths directly related to seizures fall into several categories: status epilepticus, seizure-related death, sudden unexpected death and accidents. There is an extensive literature on death in status epilepticus, which is estimated to occur in about 10% of all cases of generalized tonic clonic status. Death due to seizures is often given as an explanation used when the patient dies during or shortly after a seizure, when there is no evidence for status epilepticus and when after autopsy no other explanation can be found. An arbitrary distinction is usually made between these patients and those dying from "sudden unexpected death" but these are both likely to be to be forms of SUDEP (Sudden Unexpected Death in Epilepsy).

Common causes of death

Sudden unexpected death in epilepsy is defined as a non-traumatic unwitnessed death occurring in a patient with epilepsy who had been previously relatively healthy, for which no cause is found even after a thorough post-mortem examination. The occurrence of sudden unexpected death in epilepsy has long been recognized, being reported before the introduction of modern antiepileptic drugs. Suggested explanations for the cause of death have included suffocation during a seizure, deleterious action of antiepileptic drugs, autonomic seizures affecting the heart, and the release of endogenous opioids, although the pathophysiology (if indeed there is a single mechanism) is still unknown. *The annual mortality rate of sudden death has been variably estimated at one in two hundred to one in two thousand five hundred people with epilepsy.* The rate may be even higher among people aged 20 to 40 years, and higher still if only patients with uncontrolled seizures are selected.

Unexpected death for which no cause is found

Another possible cause of mortality and morbidity in people with epilepsy is as a result of accidents during seizures or as a consequence of a seizure. The precise extent of this problem is unknown. However, mortality rates for traumatic death are increased, indicating that accidents and trauma are a more frequent cause of death in patients with epilepsy than in the general population. There is also an increased mortality from drowning among people with epilepsy. This may occur either in the bath or while swimming. It has been suggested that the rate may be higher in countries where bathing is favored over showering, although this has never been properly investigated.

Accidents during seizures

Mortality rates also indicate that patients with epilepsy are at a higher risk of committing suicide than the general population. Patients with temporal lobe epilepsy and severe epilepsy, or epilepsy with a handicap, have a much greater risk of suicide, 25 times in the cases of temporal lobe epilepsy and five times for severe epilepsy. There seems to be some evidence that risk may decline with duration of the condition.

Higher risk of suicide

CHAPTER 4

THE ETIOLOGY AND RISK FACTORS FOR EPILEPSY

4.1   What is an "epileptic threshold"?

Epileptic seizures are produced by abnormal discharges of neurons, and may be a manifestation of many different conditions which modify neuronal function or which cause pathological changes in the brain. A plethora of environmental, genetic, pathological and physiological factors may be involved in the development of seizures. The genetic effect on susceptibility to seizures (seizure threshold) is likely to be multifactorial, and may also vary according to the stage of brain maturation. This "seizure threshold" probably determines the strength of stimulus required to generate an epileptic seizure.

Factors involved in the development of seizures

A number of precipitants for epileptic seizures are recognized. These may trigger seizures in patients with established epilepsy, and occasionally in susceptible individuals who have not had previous seizures. Among these precipitants are alcohol withdrawal, fever, head injury, infections, metabolic disturbances, photosensitivity, sleep deprivation, stress and the use of certain drugs. A variety of static or progressive pathological changes, either congenital or acquired, may predispose to seizures. In addition, a number of inherited conditions, which seem to be neurochemically determined, may express themselves solely through epileptic seizures. *It is likely that the dynamic interaction between the seizure threshold and seizure precipitants will determine an individual's propensity to have situation-related epileptic seizures, which may be isolated or recurrent, and also to develop a chronic epileptic disorder.*

Interaction between seizure threshold and precipitants

4.2   What are the most common risk factors for epilepsy?

The probable etiology depends on the age of the patient and the type of seizures. The most common acquired causes in young infants are hypoxia or birth asphyxia, perinatal intracranial trauma, metabolic disturbances, congenital

Etiology depends on age and type of seizures

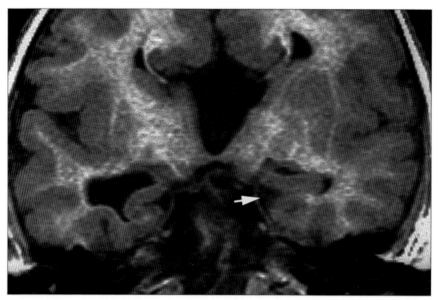

Figure 8. *MRI image in cerebral malformation: unfolded hippocampus, mesial CSF cleft and agenesis of the corpus callosum. (Courtesy of Professor John S. Duncan).*

malformations of the brain (Figure 8), and infection. In young children and adolescents, idiopathic or primary epilepsies account for the majority of seizure disorders, although trauma and infection play a role. *Febrile seizures,* which are usually short, generalized tonic clonic convulsions occurring during the early phase of a febrile disease, *are common in children aged between six months and five years, and need to be distinguished from seizures triggered by central nervous system infections causing fever,* such as meningitis and encephalitis. Unless febrile seizures are prolonged, focal, recurrent, or there is a background of neurological handicap, *the prognosis is excellent,* and it is unlikely that the child will develop chronic epilepsy.

The causes of adult onset epilepsy are very wide. Both idiopathic epilepsy and epilepsy due to birth trauma may also begin in early adulthood. Other important causes of seizures in adulthood are head injury, alcohol abuse, brain tumors and cerebrovascular disease. In developing countries, parasitic disorders such as cysticercosis and malaria may also be important causal agents for epilepsy. Brain tumors are responsible for the development of epilepsy in up to one-third of patients between the ages of 30 and 50 years. Over the age of 50, cerebrovascular disease is the most common cause of epilepsy and may be present in up to half of the patients.

Causes of adult onset epilepsy

4.3 What are the most common genetically determined epilepsies?

The idiopathic generalized or primary generalized group of conditions are probably the most common of the genetically determined epilepsies. The precise mode of inheritance for

Idiopathic generalized or primary generalized group of conditions

most of these conditions is unknown at this stage although an autosomal dominant trait is thought to be responsible in some cases.

Other inherited epileptic conditions which present with seizures as the sole clinical manifestation, including the idiopathic localization-related epilepsies (such as benign rolandic epilepsy), are also thought to be inherited in an autosomal dominant mode with incomplete penetrance.

In addition to these inherited conditions that have seizures as their main clinical expression, there are a large number of inherited disorders, most of them rare, which present as neurological or systemic illnesses of which epileptic seizures form a part. The most common of these disorders are two neurocutaneous conditions (phakomatoses): tuberous sclerosis and neurofibromatosis. Down's syndrome (trisomy 21) is also not infrequently accompanied by seizures,

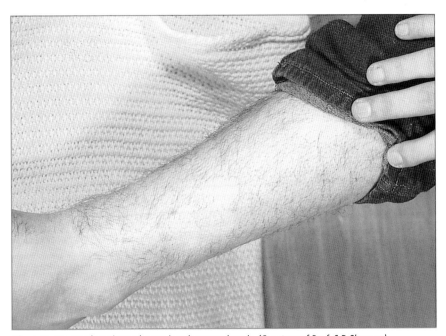

Figure 9. *Hypomelanotic patch seen in tuberous sclerosis. (Courtesy of Prof. S D Shorvon).*

particularly in later life. The progressive myoclonic epilepsies are a group of disorders characterized by the development of myoclonic and sometimes other seizures in association with other clinical manifestations which may include ataxia and progressive dementia. Rare inherited degenerative brain disorders and inborn errors of metabolism such as adrenoleukodystrophy, Alpers' disease and Tay-Sachs disease, phenylketonuria, porphyria and neuronal ceroid-lipofuscinosis may also cause seizures.

4.4   What is tuberous sclerosis?

Tuberous sclerosis (sometimes also known as adenoma sebaceum, epiloia, or Bourneville's Disease) *is inherited as an autosomal dominant condition. Linkage studies have shown loci on chromosomes 9 and 11.*

> Inherited as an autosomal dominant condition

Manifestations of the disease include partial seizures, cutaneous lesions (including facial angiofibromas, periungual fibromas, fibrous plaques of the scalp, shagreen patches and hypomelanotic areas (Figure 9)) and learning difficulties in varying degrees of severity depending on the penetrance of the gene. The most severe forms usually start in early childhood, sometimes presenting as West syndrome. In such cases severe learning difficulties are the rule. At the less severe end of the spectrum, patients may be of average intelligence with very few signs of the disease. Seizures affect more than 90% of patients and on occasion are the only clinical manifestation. The characteristic lesions seen on neuroimaging are subependymal nodules consisting of glial tissues that may be calcified ("tubers"). These are usually most prominent in the temporal lobes and are commonly situated adjacent to the ventricles. Prognosis for complete seizure control is usually guarded.

4.5   What are the features of neurofibromatosis?

Neurofibromatosis (von Recklinghausen's disease) is an autosomal dominant disease in which spots of skin hyperpigmentation (café au lait patches) are combined with

> Autosomal dominant disease

Unverricht-Lundborg disease
Lafora body disease
Neuronal ceroid lipofuscinosis
Sialidoses
Myoclonus epilepsy with ragged red fibres (MERRF)

Table 3. Some causes of progressive myoclonus epilepsy.

multiple neurofibromas arising from Schwann cells. There is a wide spectrum of severity. Mild cases may be asymptomatic, while at the other end of the spectrum major skin deformities and florid neurological manifestations are seen. Partial epileptic seizures occur in less than 10% of cases and are usually due to brain tumors such as meningioma, glioma or neurinoma, which are found in patients with neurofibromatosis at a much higher frequency than in the general population.

4.6   What are the progressive myoclonic epilepsies?

This is a heterogeneous group (Table 3) comprising several degenerative diseases that have in common the occurrence of myoclonic seizures, generalized tonic clonic convulsions and progressive intellectual deterioration, although the latter may be mild in some of the conditions. *Lafora's disease and Unverricht-Lundborg disease (familial Baltic myoclonus) are the most common disorders* in this group and both have a guarded prognosis for the control of the myoclonus and also for long-term survival. The generalized tonic clonic convulsions, however, are readily treatable with antiepileptic drugs. Mitochondrial myopathies, particularly the MERFF (Myoclonic Epilepsy and Ragged Red Fibres) and the MELAS (Myoclonic Epilepsy, Lactic Acidosis and Stroke) syndromes are also associated with progressive myoclonic epilepsy: both have a guarded prognosis.

Lafora's disease and familial Baltic myoclonus

4.7   What are the most common symptomatic or acquired epilepsies?

Common causes of symptomatic epilepsies include head trauma, birth trauma, cerebrovascular disorders, brain neoplasms, anoxia, craniotomy, brain infections including acquired immune deficiency syndrome, and some degenerative brain diseases. In developing countries, parasitic infestations such as malaria, neurocysticercosis and paragonimiasis are important causes of acquired epilepsy. It is probable that cortical dysgenesis and hippocampal sclerosis, which have been increasingly associated with chronic epilepsy, are also acquired lesions. Most epilepsies starting in adult life are symptomatic and investigations to detect the underlying etiology are mandatory.

Common causes of acquired epilepsies

4.8 What is the role of head injury in the development of symptomatic epilepsy?

Head trauma is an important cause of symptomatic partial seizures. Post-traumatic epilepsy accounts for up to 10% of all cases of epilepsy in some series. *The likelihood of developing epilepsy after head trauma depends on the severity of the injury and the presence of complicating factors, including prolonged loss of consciousness, post-traumatic amnesia of more than 30 minutes, intracranial bleeding, penetration of a missile, or a depressed skull fracture.* It is very unusual for seizures to develop unless one of these factors is present. It is thought that deposits of hemosiderin due to local bleeding may be responsible for the development of an epileptic focus at the site of injury. In the majority of cases seizures start within two years of the injury. The response to treatment is variable. Seizures occurring immediately after the injury or within the first week do not usually presage the development of chronic epilepsy.

> Severity of the injury and the presence of complicating factors

Prophylactic antiepileptic drug treatment after head injury has often been advocated in an attempt to prevent the subsequent development of epilepsy. There is, however, no clear evidence that it is effective, and *most authorities now start treatment only if seizures occur.*

4.9 What is the role of birth trauma in the development of symptomatic epilepsy?

Brain injury occurring during labor may cause symptomatic epilepsy, either as a result of direct trauma, or because of anoxia. The outcome is variable and to a large extent dependent on the severity of the injury. Birth injury was a common cause of epilepsy in the past, but with improvements in antenatal care and midwifery over the past few decades, this is no longer the case. The seizures are partial in nature, the epileptic focus being at the site of the injury. Anoxia often causes more extensive brain damage and the seizures may be generalized.

> Direct trauma or anoxia

4.10 What is the role of cerebrovascular disease in the development of symptomatic epilepsy?

Thromboembolic events and cerebral hemorrhage are important causes of symptomatic epilepsy starting in later life: they are responsible for as many as 50% of cases in this age group. Seizures are almost always partial, and usually start within a year of the

> Thromboembolic events and cerebral hemorrhage

cerebrovascular event although sometimes they may precede the stroke, suggesting previous silent ischemic episodes. Seizures occurring during or immediately after a stroke are not predictive of the late development of epilepsy. It has been estimated that **approximately 15% of people with strokes will eventually develop epileptic seizures, which are usually controlled with antiepileptic drugs.**

Vascular malformations, cerebral aneurysms, and cavernous hemangiomas (Figure 10) may also cause symptomatic epilepsy, whether or not hemorrhage has occurred. Acute subarachnoid hemorrhage may also lead to situation-related (acute symptomatic) seizures.

Sturge-Weber syndrome (encephalotrigeminal syndrome) is characterized by the presence of capillary or cavernous hemangiomas within the cutaneous distribution of the trigeminal nerve, with venous hemangiomas in the parietal, occipital and frontal regions on the same side. Either the cutaneous manifestations or the intracranial lesions may occur independently.

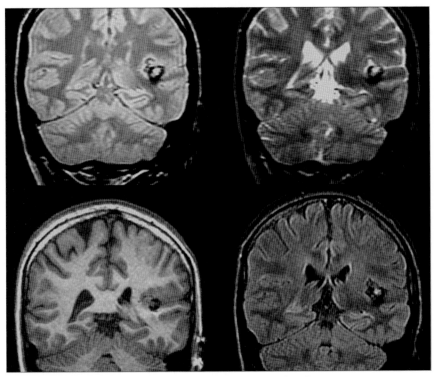

Figure 10. *MRI showing a cavernous hemangioma in a person with epilepsy. (Courtesy of Professor John S. Duncan) .*

Sturge-Weber syndrome is often associated with severe partial seizures, and the prospect for full seizure control is poor. Other neurological manifestations may also be present.

4.11 What is the role of brain tumors in the genesis of symptomatic epilepsy?

Intracranial tumors, whether benign or malignant, may cause epileptic seizures. Such tumors may arise in the brain or meninges (usually gliomas or meningiomas) or may be metastatic from a distant site. Intracranial neoplasms are responsible for about 20% of seizures starting between the ages of 30 and 50 years, and about 10% of seizures starting after the age of 50 years. The seizures are always partial in nature and are due either to mass effect or damage to surrounding cortical tissues. *The likelihood of a tumor causing seizures seems to be related to its histological type and the location.* The prognosis is largely dependent on the nature and site of the tumor.

> Intracranial tumors may cause epileptic seizures

Hamartomas, which have been classified as brain tumors by some, are occasionally found in tissue resected from patients undergoing surgery for temporal lobe epilepsy. They consist of abnormal masses of intertwined neuronal, vascular and glial tissues and are probably developmental anomalies lacking neoplastic characteristics.

4.12 Do infections of the brain cause chronic epilepsy?

Any intracranial infection, whether viral, bacterial or fungal, can cause seizures which may continue after the infection has been successfully treated. Pre- and peri-natal infections may be implicated in addition to post-natal encephalitis or meningitis. The seizures are partial, the epileptic foci occurring as a result of localized pathological changes. The severity of the epileptic disorder usually depends on the nature of the infection and the extent of the damage.

> Viral, bacterial or fungal infection may cause seizures

Meningitis is the most common intracranial infection. It is common in young children but also affects adolescents and older age groups. Epilepsy is an unusual complication of acute bacterial meningitis, occurring mainly in people given inadequate or late treatment. *Seizures are usually partial,* and the prognosis for total seizure control is in most cases guarded.

> Meningitis

Intracranial tuberculosis can cause cortical and meningeal tuberculomas which may present *with seizures sometimes developing only years after the primary infection.* The response to medical treatment is usually poor and surgery should be considered in selected cases.

Fungal infections of the central nervous system are a very rare cause of epilepsy, the most common being cryptococcosis and blastomycosis. *Cryptococcosis occurs in patients with such underlying conditions as diabetes, sarcoidosis, lymphomas and acquired immune deficiency syndrome (AIDS)* in more than 50% of cases. Blastomycosis, which affects males more than females, is prevalent in tropical and sub-tropical regions including the southeast of the United States. It should be suspected in any patient who has visited Africa or Central or South America and develops seizures in the context of an ill-defined systemic illness.

Fungal infections

Viral encephalitis, especially due to herpes, may cause epileptic seizures both during the acute phase and as a late complication. During the acute phase generalized tonic-clonic seizures are common, often resulting in status epilepticus. Seizures developing after an encephalitic process are usually partial and are often intractable to medical treatment.

Intrauterine and perinatal infections caused by such agents as toxoplasmosis, rubella and syphilis may cause extensive cortical damage, and severe partial epilepsy may result if the child survives.

A rare chronic unilateral encephalitic process known as Rasmussen's syndrome (chronic encephalitis and epilepsy) is characterized by the development of partial seizures and frequently epilepsia partialis continua, progressive hemiparesis and intellectual deterioration. Possible etiologies include a viral infection, or an autoimmune process.

Brain abscesses are rare, and are often fatal. Partial epileptic seizures develop in about three-quarters of survivors, and are usually very severe and intractable, particularly with lesions located in the frontal and temporal lobes.

4.13 In what circumstances do seizures occur in acquired immune deficiency syndrome?

Involvement of the central nervous system eventually occurs in the majority of people developing AIDS. It may take the form of opportunistic infection or neoplastic lesions.

> HIV testing should be considered in patients with risk factors

An encephalopathy that seems to be caused by the human immunodeficiency virus (HIV) itself has also been recognized. Any of these conditions may present with epileptic seizures, either as the initial manifestation or late in the disease. Seizures due to opportunistic infections and neoplasms are usually of a partial nature, while those due to HIV encephalopathy are usually generalized tonic-clonic convulsions. The diagnosis, particularly when a seizure is the first manifestation, may be difficult, and *HIV testing should be considered in patients with risk factors.*

4.14 Which parasitic infections may be associated with epilepsy?

Epilepsy may occur in the course of a number of parasitic disorders, including neurocysticercosis (due to *Taenia solium*), malaria (*Plasmodium falciparum*), schistosomiasis (*Schistosoma japonicum*), paragonimiasis or endemic haemoptysis (*Paragonimus westermani*), toxocariasis (*Toxocara canis*), onchocerciasis or river blindness (*Onchocerca volvulus*) and American trypanosomiasis or Chagas' disease (*Trypanosoma cruzi*). *Such infections may be responsible for the high incidence of epilepsy in some parts of the tropical world.* The most common to be associated with epilepsy are neurocysticercosis and falciparum malaria.

Neurocysticercosis is the most common acquired cause of epilepsy in some developing countries, particularly in Latin America. This occurs when man becomes the intermediate host for *Taenia solium* (the pork tapeworm) through the ingestion of eggs contained in human feces. Cysts containing an embryo may emerge in any area of the cerebrum, ventricles or subarachnoid space of the infested patient (Figure 11), leading to a variety of neurological signs including partial seizures, which may sometimes be the only manifestation. Prognosis is variable and usually depends on the number and location of the cysts. Neurocysticercosis should be suspected in any individual developing partial seizures who has lived in or visited an endemic area.

Cerebral malaria, which is the most important complication of falciparum malaria, may first present as status epilepticus. It carries a high mortality and

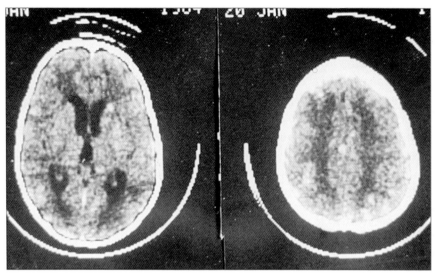

Figure 11. CT scan showing neurocysticercosis. (Courtesy of Dr Paulo Bittencourt).

morbidity. Survivors often have partial seizures that respond poorly to treatment with antiepileptic drugs.

4.15 What is the risk of epilepsy after craniotomy?

Neurosurgical procedures involving the supratentorial region are associated with the development of epileptic seizures in about 10% of cases. The incidence, however, varies depending on the location and the condition for which the craniotomy was performed. In patients with uncomplicated aneurysm surgery it may be as low as 5%, while it can be as high as 90% following surgery for cerebral abscess. The seizures are usually partial, and occur within the first year in the majority of cases. There is no evidence that prophylactic antiepileptic drug treatment after craniotomy reduces the risk of developing epilepsy, although it is sometimes advocated.

> The development of epilepsy may occur after about 10% of neurosurgical procedures involving the supratentorial region

4.16 Can epilepsy occur in degenerative brain diseases?

Epilepsy may sometimes complicate degenerative brain conditions such as Alzheimer's disease, Huntington's chorea, striatonigral degeneration and Jakob-Creutzfeld disease. Patients with Alzheimer's disease are at considerably increased risk of developing epileptic seizures, with as many as 20% of patients being affected.

4.17   What proportion of patients with multiple sclerosis develop seizures?

Epileptic seizures occur in about 4% of people with multiple sclerosis and are rarely the first manifestation of the condition. Seizures are usually partial in nature although generalized tonic clonic convulsions may also occur. *The prognosis for seizure control is usually good* although the overall prognosis is that of the background condition, that is, highly varied and unpredictable.

> 4% of people with multiple sclerosis develop epileptic seizures

4.18   What is the risk of epilepsy following vaccination?

An allergic reaction to vaccine components very occasionally leads to an acute encephalopathy which may cause acute symptomatic seizures and also result in chronic epilepsy. Such a reaction has been reported following vaccination against rabies, smallpox and whooping-cough (pertussis). *It is however, extremely rare, and is becoming even more uncommon as more purified and less antigenic vaccines are used.*

> Allergic reaction may lead to acute encephalopathy

It is important to note that *the incidence of epilepsy is at its highest in early childhood,* the age at which most vaccinations are carried out, and therefore *some children will develop seizures in temporal association with vaccination by coincidence.* Other children experience a febrile reaction to some vaccinations and may have a febrile seizure as a result, without long-term sequelae.

The presence of a history of epileptic seizures or of a family history of epilepsy in a child is no longer considered a contraindication to immunization, since the risk of the condition for which the inoculation is being given is greater than that of vaccination.

4.19   Under what circumstances does anoxia cause epilepsy?

Anoxia sufficiently severe to cause epilepsy is probably most common in the perinatal period. It is usually associated with severe morbidity, with epileptic seizures being a common manifestation. Anoxia may also occur in the course of a cardiac or respiratory arrest, and may be followed by the development of chronic myoclonic seizures.

4.20 What are cortical dysplasias?

Errors in neuronal migration during embryogenesis may result in cortical dysplasias or dysgenesis: in an analogy with the skin these would constitute the "bumps and blemishes" of the brain. Cortical dysgenesis was until recently considered to be rare: however, with the development of modern neuroimaging techniques, particularly high-resolution magnetic resonance scanning, it is being recognized with increasing frequency. Cortical dysplasias can be divided into four broad categories: gyral abnormalities, heterotopias, focal cortical dysplasias including microdysgenesis, and proliferative dysgenesis.

Errors in neuronal migration during embryogenesis

Gyral abnormalities include agyria or lissencephaly (absence of gyri over the whole brain), schizencephaly (Figure 12, with 3-D reconstruction Figure 13) (in which clefts extend from the cortex to the ventricular surface) and localized areas of macrogyria (Figure 14) or polymicrogyria (Figure 15). Heterotopias consist of bands or nodules of normal neurons which are located incorrectly, usually subcortically (Figures 16, 17). Focal cortical dysplasias and microdysgenesis are characterized by clusters of abnormal neurons usually positioned in aberrant locations (Figure 18). Among the proliferative dysgeneses are dysembryoplastic neuroepithelial tumors (Figure 19). These are benign congenital lesions which are easily confused with low-grade gliomas. They are predominantly cortical, often multi-nodular, may contain cystic components and have associated areas of cortical dysgenesis.

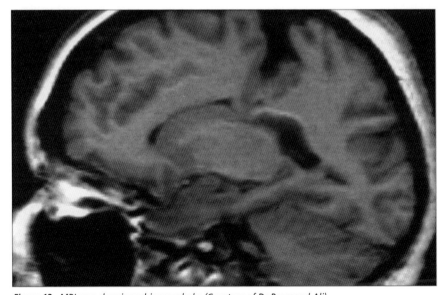

Figure 12. *MRI scan showing schizencephaly. (Courtesy of Dr Raymond Ali).*

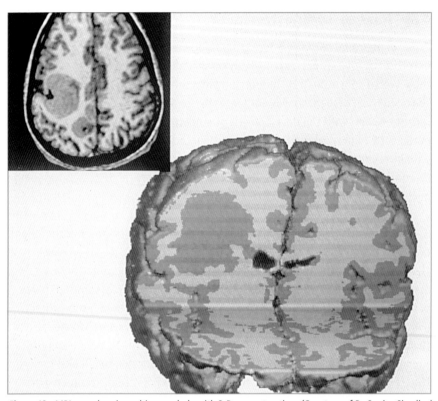

Figure 13. *MRI scan showing schizencephaly with 3-D reconstruction. (Courtesy of Dr Sanjay Sisodiya).*

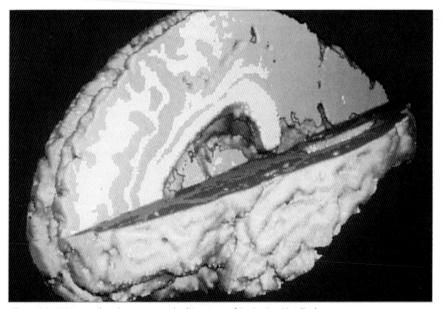

Figure 14. *MRI scan showing macrogyria. (Courtesy of Dr Sanjay Sisodiya).*

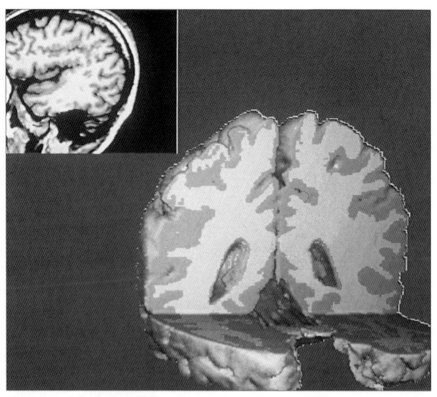

Figure 15. *MRI scan showing polymicrogyria. (Courtesy of Dr Sanjay Sisodiya).*

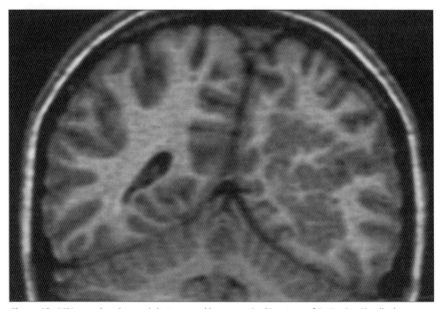

Figure 16. *MRI scan showing occipitotemporal heterotopia. (Courtesy of Dr Sanjay Sisodiya).*

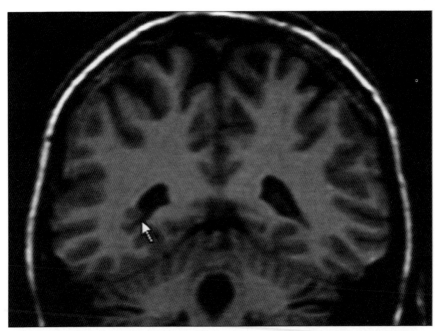

Figure 17. *MRI scan showing nodular subependymal heterotopia. (Courtesy of Dr Raymond Ali).*

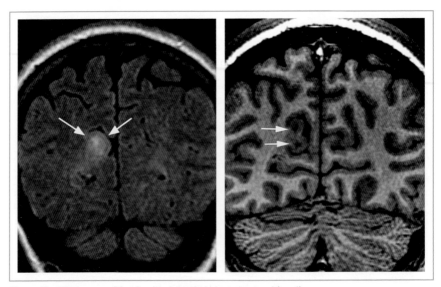

Figure 18. *MRI images of focal cortical dysplasia in a person with epilepsy. (Courtesy of Professor John Duncan).*

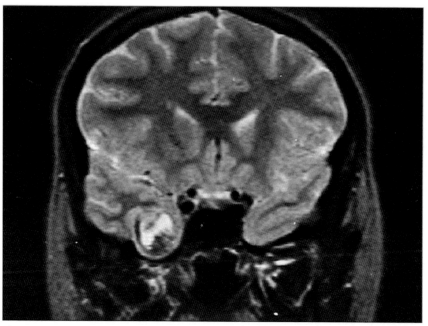

Figure 19. *MRI scan showing dysembryoplastic neuroepithelial tumor. (Courtesy of Dr Sanjay Sisodiya).*

The etiology of cortical dysplasias is unknown at this stage, but potential causes are thought to include intrauterine infection, genetic syndromes, maternal illness or exposure to toxins at 8-16 weeks of gestation when neuronal migration occurs, or insults occurring in the last trimester of gestation when gyral formation takes place.

4.21 What is the association between cortical dysplasias and epilepsy?

Cortical dysplasias are increasingly being recognized as a major cause of chronic epilepsy. It has been estimated that at post-mortem examination, cortical dysplasias are found in 25-60% of

Major cause of chronic epilepsy

the brains of patients with epilepsy, compared with 8% of control brains. The majority of these patients had been classified as having cryptogenic epilepsy.

Epilepsy associated with cortical dysplasias often presents in the first decade of life but may be delayed as late as the second decade or even beyond. Except when major abnormalities are present, the intellectual development of patients is usually within the normal range. Many patients with cortical dysplasias give a history of other factors which may have contributed to the development of epilepsy, and some people with lesions never develop epilepsy; it may be that a second insult is required to trigger the seizures in a proportion of cases.

Seizures are usually partial but some patients have only generalized seizures. Response to antiepileptic drug treatment is very variable. Patients with dysembryoplastic neuroepithelial tumors may benefit from surgery.

4.22 What is hippocampal sclerosis?

Hippocampal sclerosis (also known as Ammon's horn sclerosis, temporal horn sclerosis or mesial temporal sclerosis) *is the most common lesion identified in pathological specimens of patients with temporal lobe epilepsy who have undergone temporal lobectomy.* It consists of atrophic changes with a variable degree of cell loss and gliosis involving part or the whole of the hippocampus. It is usually unilateral and can be identified by high-resolution magnetic resonance imaging (Figure 20). Minor asymmetry of the hippocampi, which may suggest sclerosis in the smaller hippocampus, is difficult to determine by visual

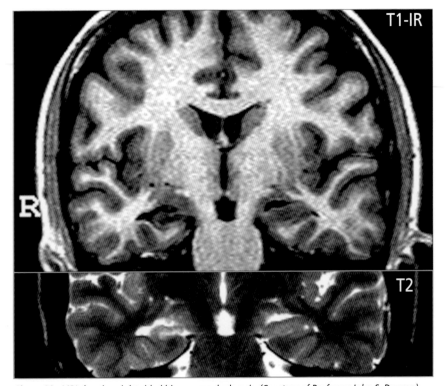

Figure 20. MRI showing right-sided hippocampal sclerosis. (Courtesy of Professor John S. Duncan).

inspection, but can be quantified using MRI-assisted volumetric measurement. Temporal lobe epilepsy with hippocampal sclerosis is strongly associated with a history of prolonged febrile convulsions in childhood.

4.23 What is the relationship between hippocampal sclerosis and epilepsy?

This ongoing controversy in the epilepsy world questions whether hippocampal sclerosis results from epileptic activity, or whether it precedes the epileptic condition and represents the cause of the seizures. There are some indications that prolonged febrile convulsions in childhood may cause hippocampal damage and the subsequent development of temporal lobe epilepsy, but this has not yet been proven conclusively. *There is, however, no doubt about the link between severe intractable temporal lobe seizures and hippocampal sclerosis.* Resection of the atrophic area, when possible, is associated with a very good surgical outcome with complete seizure control in over 70% of cases.

4.24 Which intrauterine conditions cause seizures?

Conditions that affect the child while still in the mother's womb may cause epilepsy as a result of brain damage or malformation. Intrauterine infections (see above) are an example of this, as is erythroblastosis fetalis, an uncommon disease caused by incompatibility between the blood of the fetus and the mother. Cortical dysplasias are also thought to be caused during the intrauterine period (see over page).

Conditions which result in brain damage or malformation

4.25 Which drugs can trigger seizures?

A number of drugs have been associated with the precipitation of seizures in patients with epilepsy. Most of these drugs may also trigger situation-related seizures in individuals with a low seizure threshold. Examples of such drugs include some antidepressants, antibiotics, anesthetic agents, antimalarial drugs, beta-blockers, bronchodilators, chemotherapeutic agents, iodinated contrast media and neuroleptic agents. Some recreational drugs such as alcohol, amphetamine and cocaine are also associated with seizures.

4.26 Which systemic diseases cause epileptic seizures?

Epileptic seizures may complicate many systemic diseases, usually as a result of metabolic disturbances. Any conditions which cause imbalance in the extracellular distribution of sodium, potassium, calcium, magnesium or phosphate have the potential to produce seizures. Hypoglycemia occurring either in patients taking insulin or other hypoglycemic agents, or patients with insulinoma may also present in this way. Other conditions that may be complicated by seizures include acute liver failure, eclampsia, and both acute and chronic renal failure. In the majority of cases, however, these are acute symptomatic attacks and therefore do not constitute epilepsy even if they are recurrent.

Epileptic seizures may complicate systemic diseases

4.27 What is reflex epilepsy?

When there is a clear-cut precipitant for epileptic seizures in a given patient, and if seizures only occur as a result of the triggering factor, the condition is referred to as reflex epilepsy. The most common reflex seizures are photically-induced. About 50% of patients with photosensitivity will only have seizures as a response to visual stimuli. Other rarer forms of reflex epilepsy include reading epilepsy, writing epilepsy, startle-induced epilepsy, arithmetic-induced seizures and musicogenic seizures.

Patients who have seizures precipitated by a particular stimulus but who also have spontaneous seizures should not be classified as having reflex epilepsy.

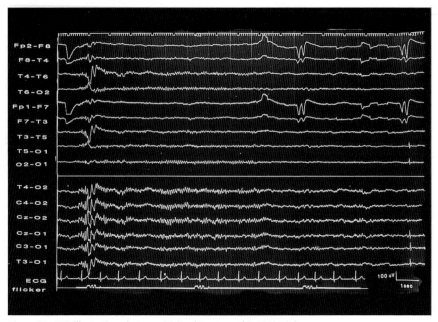

Figure 21. *EEG illustrating photosensitivity. (Courtesy of Dr Li Li Min).*

4.28 What is photosensitivity?

In people with idiopathic generalized epilepsy, photosensitivity is a common finding. *Patients with a photosensitive response account for about 2-3% of all people with epilepsy, the proportion being higher in patients aged between five and 19 years.* The trait is genetically determined, and may be asymptomatic throughout or present as a medical problem because of epileptic seizures.

2-3% of all people with epilepsy have photosensitive responses

It may only be detected by an EEG (Figure 21) although it should be suspected in patients giving a history of seizures precipitated by flashing lights. Potential precipitants of seizures in photosensitive patients include lights from natural sources such as sunlight passing through trees in a road or reflection in an aquatic surface, or from artificial sources like flashing lights, computer or television screens. *There is no evidence to suggest that flashing lights cause the development of the photosensitive trait, merely that they can trigger seizures in people harboring this trait.* Photosensitivity is a clinically heterogeneous phenomenon, and photosensitive subjects show wide variation in their susceptibility to seizures.

No evidence that flashing lights cause photosensitive trait

4.29 What is catamenial epilepsy?

Catamenial epilepsy is the term used to describe seizures occurring in women in association with the menstrual period (either immediately preceding or during menstruation). Suggested causes include hormonal imbalance, water retention and electrolyte disturbances associated with menses. Catamenial epilepsy is discussed further in Chapter 9.

4.30 When should epilepsy be termed cryptogenic?

The term "cryptogenic epilepsy" is used when no putative etiology is identified for what is presumed to be a symptomatic or acquired epileptic condition. Currently about 30% of patients do not have an identifiable cause for their seizures but this proportion is rapidly decreasing as advances in neuroimaging, particularly in magnetic resonance imaging, are made.

No putative etiology is identified

The term cryptogenic epilepsy is sometimes used interchangeably with idiopathic epilepsy. This should be avoided, however, as the term idiopathic epilepsy should be reserved for those inherited conditions in which seizures occur as the only manifestation of the disorder.

CHAPTER 5

THE PATHOPHYSIOLOGY OF EPILEPSY

5.1 What is the pathognomonic lesion of epilepsy?

Epilepsy differs from most neurological conditions in having no pathognomonic lesion. Epileptic seizures which are associated with structural abnormalities, however, may have histopathological findings (such as heterotopias or vascular lesions) which are pathognomonic for that condition, rather than for the epilepsy itself. No specific histopathological or histochemical abnormality has yet been identified which is associated with the potential to cause epileptic discharges.

No pathognomonic lesion

At the neuronal level, a variety of different electrical or chemical stimuli can lead to the development of seizures in a normal brain. *The hallmark of epilepsy, regardless of the type or etiology, is a rather rhythmic and repetitive hypersynchronous discharge of neurons, either localized to a particular area of the cerebral cortex or generalized throughout the cortex.* This can usually be demonstrated on an EEG. Despite this, no unifying theory for all aspects of human epileptogenesis has yet been advanced. It is likely that several different pathophysiological mechanisms are responsible for the onset, maintenance and spread of seizures, and these may vary according to the type of epileptic disorder.

Rhythmic and repetitive hypersynchronous discharge of neurons

A large number of studies using experimental models of epilepsy and functional studies of the brain in vivo are ongoing. It is hoped that enough evidence will eventually emerge to provide a better understanding of the pathophysiology and biochemistry of human epileptogenesis.

5.2 What are experimental models of epilepsy?

Experimental models of epilepsy are standardized methods for producing epilepsy in experimental animals. They are classified into acute and chronic models. The former refers to models which are based on the systemic administration or topical application of convulsant materials or sudden insults such as electrical stimulation that will induce epileptic seizures. Chronic models are based on seizures occurring spontaneously in animals (such as baboons, gerbils and beagle dogs) inbred to produce a genetic predisposition to epilepsy or caused by permanent structural lesions or the repetitive electrical stimulation of areas of the brain.

5.3 Can the findings of animal models be extrapolated to human epilepsy?

Most of what is assumed about human epileptogenesis is extrapolated from research carried out in experimental animal models of epilepsy. These models have never been properly validated and the relevance of these results to human epilepsy is therefore difficult to assess. *There are, however, some electrophysiological similarities between the animal models and human epilepsy,* and some findings from animal models have been confirmed in vivo. This gives some credence to the assumption that findings from these models can be applied to human epilepsy.

Electrophysiological similarities between the animal models and human epilepsy

5.4 What is the role of neurotransmitters in the genesis of epilepsy?

Neurons are interconnected in a complex network in which each individual neuron is linked through synapses with hundreds of others. *A small electrical discharge in a neuron causes the release of a neurotransmitter substance at the synaptic level, thus enabling communication between neurons.* Neurotransmitters are of two types: inhibitory and excitatory. A discharging neuron may thus either excite or inhibit neurons associated with it. An excited neuron will activate the next neuron whereas an inhibited neuron will not. In this manner, information is transmitted throughout the central nervous system.

Enables communication through neurons

A whole array of neurotransmitters seems to exist and it is quite possible that some have not yet been identified. *The most important known inhibitory neurotransmitter is gamma-amino-butyric acid (GABA) of which several forms have already been recognized.* Excitatory transmission seems to be dependent on amino acids, of which glutamate and aspartate are the most well-known at this stage. It is possible that either a lack or an excess of neurotransmitters of either category may play a part in the disruption of the processes of neuronal transmission and thus lead to epileptic seizures.

Gamma-amino-butyric acid

5.5 How does an epileptic seizure start?

A normal neuron discharges repetitively at a low baseline frequency and it is the integrated electrical activity generated by the neurons of the superficial layers of the cortex, which is recorded in a normal EEG. If neurons are damaged or suffer a chemical or metabolic insult, a change in the pattern of discharges may develop. In the case of *partial epilepsy, regular low frequency discharges are replaced by bursts of high frequency discharges usually followed by periods of inactivity.*

Bursts of high frequency

A single neuron discharging in an abnormal manner is usually of no clinical significance: it is only when a whole population of neurons discharge synchronously in an abnormal way that an epileptic seizure may be triggered. Little is known about the precise mechanisms which lead to this synchronisation and consequently to seizure onset. The abnormal discharge may remain localized or it may spread to adjacent areas recruiting more neurons as it spreads. It may also generalize throughout the brain via cortical and subcortical routes including callosal and thalamocortical pathways. The area from which the original discharge originates is known as the epileptic focus.

In idiopathic generalized absences the mechanisms are even less understood but they are probably different. The discharges are thought to arise from, or be modulated by, the thalamus rather than from the cerebral cortex and the way they spread is also likely to be different.

5.6 Why are seizures self-limited?

It is not known why epileptic seizures cease spontaneously in the vast majority of cases. It is likely that inhibitory substances are released in the cortex and terminate the seizure. Recent speculation has centered on the role of endogenous opioids in such a process.

5.7 Does ictal activity cause brain damage?

Another controversial area in epilepsy is whether seizure activity may itself cause neuronal damage or functional changes. It has been suggested that chronic epileptic discharges may lead to secondary epileptogenesis (kindling). Evidence for this in some experimental models of partial seizures is convincing but similar evidence is lacking in humans, in whom the hypothesis is difficult to test.

Chronic epileptic discharges may lead to secondary epileptogenesis

It is thought that short, uncomplicated seizures cause no permanent or progressive neurological dysfunction in humans. Prolonged generalized tonic clonic status epilepticus is associated with a high neurological morbidity and may result in permanent brain damage. It is, however, probable that this is at least in part due to systemic factors such as hypoperfusion, hypoxia, acidosis and other metabolic disturbances associated with status.

CHAPTER 6

THE DIAGNOSIS AND INVESTIGATION OF EPILEPSY

6.1   How is the diagnosis of epilepsy made?

The diagnosis of epilepsy is clinical, and rests on the description of the seizure provided by the patient and an eye-witness. The report of the eye-witness is of great importance, especially if there is any impairment of consciousness during the seizure. The diagnosis of epilepsy involves not only confirming that the events experienced are seizures, but also the identification, where possible, of the underlying cause, and categorization of the seizure type(s) and epilepsy syndrome according to the classifications of the International League Against Epilepsy [1-3].

Issues which should be addressed include the nature of the aura, if present; the ictal manifestations themselves; and the presence or absence of post-ictal confusion, drowsiness or headache. *Any precipitating factors should be sought. A full medical (including neurological) history should be taken in addition to details of previous psychiatric problems, and a family history.* The patient should be asked particularly whether he or she has ever had febrile convulsions, significant head injury, encephalitis or meningitis, and whether his or her birth was normal.

> Clinical diagnosis

> Detailed medical history

6.2   With what conditions may epilepsy be confused?

There are many disorders involving alteration of consciousness, or focal neurological symptoms, which may be confused with epileptic seizures: these are summarized in Table 4. The conditions most commonly mistaken for epileptic seizures are syncope and non-epileptic seizures (this term is commonly used to describe seizures which have a psychological cause, but may also include other non-epileptic events).

> Non-epileptic seizures

SYNCOPE

Syncope may be due to a number of causes, including strong emotion, prolonged standing, particularly if the ambient temperature is hot, cardiac arrhythmias, and pain. It rarely occurs in patients who are recumbent. It is almost invariably preceded by a warning in which the patient may feel faint and sometimes nauseous, his or her vision may become blurred, and hearing may become muffled. To an observer, the patient appears pale, and may sweat profusely. Consciousness is then usually lost and the patient falls to the floor. Quick recovery occurs provided the patient is not raised to an upright position. Incontinence and injury may sometimes occur. Eye-rolling and brief jerking movements (usually appearing as multifocal myoclonic jerks) may also be seen, particularly if the patient is raised, and if they are maintained in the upright position, a tonic clonic seizure may occur. Afterwards, the patient may feel nauseated and shaky but not confused or drowsy. *The features of cardiac syncope can often differ* in that the patient may have no warning, and does not necessarily recover on lying down.

Syncope	Movement disorders
Psychogenic non-epileptic seizures	Narcolepsy
Panic attacks	Transient ischemic attacks
Hyperventilation	Migraine
Episodic dyscontrol syndrome	Transient global amnesia
Breath-holding attacks	Hypoglycemia
Night terrors	Vertigo

Table 4. Conditions which may be confused with epilepsy.

PSYCHOGENIC NON-EPILEPTIC SEIZURES

This term is used to describe non-epileptic seizures of psychological origin (rather than the term "psychogenic seizures", which is used by some authors to describe genuine epileptic seizures induced by the patient at will, for example, by fluttering the eyelids in the case of photosensitive epilepsy). Other terms which have been used to describe this condition are non-epileptic attack disorder (NEAD), pseudoseizures, and hysterical seizures. *It is common experience in specialized*

Syncope and psychogenic non-epileptic seizures

centers that around 20% of patients admitted to hospital with a diagnosis of intractable epilepsy do not have epileptic seizures. However, psychogenic non-epileptic seizures (PNES) also occur not infrequently in people with epilepsy.

PNES are more common in women. There may be a past or family history of psychiatric disorder, sometimes including unexplained neurological dysfunction or previous attempted suicide. The attacks tend to start in the teens or twenties, and do not usually respond to the introduction of antiepileptic drugs, unlike genuine epileptic seizures. The attacks may include thrashing or flailing of the limbs, sometimes with pelvic thrusting and opisthotonus: in other patients, they may take the appearance of a "swoon", in which the patient lies perfectly still. If the attacks have the appearance of generalized tonic clonic seizures, serial measurements of serum prolactin levels after a seizure may sometimes help in the differentiation from genuine epileptic attacks. Psychogenic "status epilepticus" may also occur in patients with PNES, who are thus at risk of receiving large doses of antiepileptic medication even to the extent that assisted ventilation may be used, with all the attendant hazards.

PANIC ATTACKS

Panic attacks are common in people with anxiety states. The patient feels anxious, and this feeling is accompanied by such physical symptoms as palpitations, dyspnea, sweating, trembling and abdominal discomfort. Usually it is possible to distinguish such attacks from the history, but occasionally seizures of temporal lobe origin may have similar symptomatology.

HYPERVENTILATION

Periods of stress

This is another common disorder which is not infrequently confused with epilepsy. Attacks usually occur during periods of stress. Hyperventilation causes a feeling of dizziness and sometimes even altered awareness or loss of consciousness. The patient may also complain of chest pain, dyspnea, blurred vision, paraesthesias, muscle cramps and fatigue.

EPISODIC DYSCONTROL SYNDROME

Rage attacks, often occurring apparently out of character, are sometimes attributed to epilepsy. In practice, however, rage occurring in the context of epileptic seizures is rare, unprovoked, and usually undirected.

BREATH-HOLDING ATTACKS

These occur in children, usually under the age of six years, and are commonly mistaken for seizures, although if witnessed, diagnosis should be possible from the history of precipitating factors. Cyanotic breath-holding attacks occur when the child is frustrated or angry. A period of crying is followed by the cessation of breathing. Cyanosis follows and the child becomes limp and unresponsive; sometimes trembling or a few clonic movements occur. Unresponsiveness usually persists for about two minutes and is followed by rapid recovery. Pallid breath-holding attacks often follow minor head-trauma. The child may not cry, but abruptly loses consciousness and becomes limp. Clonic movements are common as a result of cerebral hypoxia, but recovery is fairly rapid.

Occur in younger children

DAY-DREAMING

Innocent day-dreaming may occasionally be mistaken for true absence attacks, but can be distinguished by the fact that the child can be easily alerted, and by the absence of postural changes or automatisms.

SLEEP PHENOMENA

There are several sleep phenomena which may be confused with epileptic seizures. Sleep-walking is common in children, and is characterized by automatic behavior (which does not always involve the patient getting out of bed) during non-REM sleep. Night-terrors are also common in children and likewise occur in deep slow-wave sleep. The child suddenly sits up, crying or screaming, sweating and with dilated pupils. Eventually the child calms down and normal sleep is resumed. Afterwards however, there is amnesia for the attack. It is less common for nightmares to be mistaken for seizures. *Hypnic jerks occur in the majority of people from time to time,* and take the form of a single jerk occurring in the early stages of sleep, often accompanied by a falling sensation and causing awakening. Periodic movements of sleep occur in later life and are characterized by the presence of repetitive rhythmic leg movements, often with dorsiflexion of the foot and extension of the toes. Sleep apnea may rarely also be mistaken for epilepsy. Paroxysmal nocturnal dystonias, which at one time were considered to be an uncommon movement disorder of sleep, are now recognized to be due to frontal lobe seizures.

May be confused with epileptic seizures

Narcolepsy is a condition in which sudden irresistible attacks of daytime sleepiness occur. Cataplexy is characterized by sudden falls as a result of postural tone loss; either type of attack may occasionally be confused with epileptic seizures.

MIGRAINE

There are several reasons why migraine attacks may be confused with epileptic seizures. Syncope may occur during the course of the migraine, particularly when vomiting occurs. Basilar migraine may present with loss of consciousness, often in association with other symptoms and followed by headache, causing confusion with epileptic seizures. The accompanying brainstem symptoms and a family history of migraine may help in their differentiation. *Migraine preceded by visual or sensory disturbances may also be mistaken for partial epilepsies.* It should be noted that interictal paroxysmal EEG phenomena may be seen in migraine.

Migraine preceded by visual or sensory disturbances

TRANSIENT ISCHEMIC ATTACKS

Last longer than epileptic seizures

Transient ischemic attacks may produce weakness and sensory symptoms; it is the latter which usually cause confusion with epileptic seizures. *Transient ischemic attacks usually last longer than epileptic seizures, and there is rarely loss of consciousness.* Sensory phenomena in epilepsy may spread in the manner of a Jacksonian march. This is not usually the case in transient ischemic attacks. In addition, transient ischemic attacks are more likely to involve loss of function (such as weakness, numbness or loss of vision), whereas seizures are more likely to involve positive phenomena, such as jerking or paraesthesias. However, this is only a rough guide, and exceptions may occur, for example "limb shaking TIAs" as a hemodynamic phenomenon of severe carotid artery disease.

TRANSIENT GLOBAL AMNESIA

Transient global amnesia is a condition usually occurring in middle-aged or older people. Most often this occurs as an isolated episode lasting several hours, in which the patient is unable to remember. He or she remains alert and communicative throughout this period, but may repeatedly ask the same question. *Except for amnesia for the duration of the episode, recovery afterwards is complete.* The cause of transient global amnesia remains unclear.

Migraine, epilepsy and cerebrovascular disease have been suggested, but in the majority of people epilepsy is not implicated. Where it is the cause of memory loss (transient epileptic amnesia), the attacks are usually short-lived and recurrent, often occur on awakening in the morning, and are associated with other features of epilepsy (for example, orofacial or manual automatisms or other seizure types, EEG abnormalities, or their response to antiepileptic drugs).

MOVEMENT DISORDERS

A variety of movement disorders may on occasion be mistaken for seizures, although the distinction is not usually difficult. *Tics and chorea may sometimes be confused with myoclonus.* Paroxysmal choreoathetosis is a familial disorder characterized by repeated episodes of dystonia or choreoathetosis, unaccompanied by loss of consciousness. Despite the absence of EEG abnormalities during the attacks, the condition often responds to antiepileptic medication. In paroxysmal kinesigenic choreoathetosis the attacks, which are short-lived, are precipitated by sudden movement. Tonic spasms similar to those seen in paroxysmal chorea are also sometimes seen in multiple sclerosis.

> *Tics and chorea may be confused with myoclonus*

Paroxysmal familial ataxia is an inherited condition in which episodes of ataxia lasting up to 30 minutes may occur, without other accompaniments. *It has been reported in people of Mediterranean origin,* and it is important to recognize since it may have an excellent response to acetazolamide.

> *Paroxysmal familial ataxia may respond to acetazolamide*

HYPOGLYCEMIA

Hypoglycemia most commonly affects people with diabetes, and in particular, those taking insulin or oral hypoglycemic agents. Occasionally, however, it is due to insulinoma. Hypoglycemia normally first produces autonomic changes, including pallor, sweating, and tachycardia, and these may be recognized by the patient who can then take appropriate action. If autonomic changes do not occur, or if there is no warning, coma ensues, and genuine seizures may eventually supervene.

VERTIGO

Vertigo has many causes but is often paroxysmal, and as a result, is sometimes misdiagnosed as epilepsy. Very occasionally, vertigo may itself be a symptom of an epileptic seizure, particularly in the case of parietal lobe epilepsy. Care should be taken over the interpretation of the use of the word "dizzy" by patients, which may variously serve to mean vertiginous, light-headed, or vague.

Misdiagnosed as epilepsy

6.3 Are there any particular signs which should be sought in the examination of patients with epilepsy?

All patients developing seizures should have a complete general and neurological examination. Specific signs which should be checked include the presence of any cutaneous stigmata which may indicate the cause of the epilepsy (for example café au lait spots, adenoma sebaceum, or trigeminal capillary hemangiomas, suggesting the possibility of neurofibromatosis, tuberous sclerosis, and Sturge-Weber syndrome respectively). *Focal neurological deficits suggesting the presence of a structural lesion should be assiduously sought.* Abnormalities may be subtle, for example, impairment of fine finger movements. The patient should also be examined for any evidence of hemiatrophy, indicating a cerebral lesion occurring early in life.

Focal neurological deficits should be sought

6.4 Which patients, if any, require investigation after a single seizure?

The aims of investigation are to increase diagnostic accuracy and clarify the seizure type, and most importantly to identify the cause of the seizures. An indication of prognosis may also be obtained if a specific cause or epilepsy syndrome, such as benign epilepsy of childhood with centrotemporal spikes, is identified. It has been argued that seizures occurring as a result of tumor or other sinister cause are likely to recur, and that investigation may be deferred until the occurrence of a second seizure. However, the identification of an underlying cause or syndrome may have implications for prognosis or treatment, and *investigation should therefore be carried out at an early stage in all patients developing seizures.*

6.5 Which investigations should be performed in patients developing seizures?

As has been stated above, *the diagnosis of epilepsy is clinical, and depends mainly on the description of the attack.* EEG should only be carried out in those patients in whom there is a strong suspicion of epilepsy. In such patients, the finding of obvious epileptic abnormalities in the EEG lends weight to the diagnosis, and the seizure type may also be clarified. The use of the EEG is described in more detail below.

Epileptic abnormalities in the EEG

The history and examination not infrequently give a clue to etiology particularly in the case of acute symptomatic or situation-related seizures (seizures occurring in the context of a metabolic disturbance, drugs, or other acute insult to the brain, such as head injury, stroke or infection). Seizures can occur with disorders of sodium, calcium, magnesium, and glucose metabolism, in renal failure and acute hepatic failure, and occasionally with thyroid disease. Biochemical tests for these disorders, in addition to full blood count, erythrocyte sedimentation rate (ESR), and syphilis serology, should be performed as clinically indicated. However, routine screening in otherwise fit people has a low yield.

Blackouts or dizzy spells due to cardiac arrhythmias may be confused with seizures. An electrocardiogram or 24 hour cardiac monitoring should be performed where appropriate, particularly in the elderly. For those patients in whom a cardiac cause seems likely, referral for cardiac assessment and investigation should be made. In patients having occasional attacks in whom a cardiac cause is suspected but cannot otherwise be confirmed, the use of an implantable loop recorder may be considered.

In children, the possibility of inborn errors of metabolism should be considered (Table 5). Special investigation is only necessary when there are specific

Birth asphyxia
Infection
Metabolic disorders (including hypoglycemia, hypocalcemia, pyridoxine deficiency)
Intracranial hemorrhage
Maternal drug use
Benign idiopathic neonatal convulsions ("fifth day fits")
Benign familial neonatal convulsions
Other

Table 5. Causes of neonatal seizures.

features to suggest such a condition, and should be tailored according to the clinical picture.

The major causes of neonatal seizures are shown in Table 5. The proportion of seizures due to each cause has differed in various studies, but the largest single cause of neonatal seizures (30-50%) is considered to be birth asphyxia. However, in some surveys up to one-third of neonatal seizures have been benign idiopathic neonatal convulsions ("fifth day fits"). The cause of the seizures may be suggested by the history and examination, and investigations need to be tailored to the individual infant.

Birth asphyxia is considered the largest single cause of neonatal seizures

6.6 How does an EEG help in making the diagnosis of epilepsy?

The diagnosis of epilepsy can neither be made nor refuted on the basis of an interictal EEG, though epileptic abnormalities make the diagnosis more likely. Approximately 35% of patients with epilepsy show interictal epileptiform activity in all routine waking recordings, 15% do not show interictal epileptiform abnormalities even after multiple EEGs, and the remainder (50-55%) show epileptiform activity in some but not all recordings.

Fewer than 1% of normal subjects, with no clinical evidence of epilepsy and without other cerebral disease, have focal or generalized spike or polyspike and wave abnormalities on the EEG, although between 10 and 15% of the population may have minor non-specific abnormalities. People undergoing EEG examinations because of other complaints, but without clinical evidence of seizures, have an incidence of epileptiform abnormalities of 2-3%, as do those taking major tranquillizers or antidepressants. In those with learning difficulties the incidence may be as high as 30%.

6.7 If the initial EEG is normal, are there other investigations which may be helpful in making the diagnosis?

If epilepsy is suggested clinically, corroborative evidence may be derived from an EEG obtained during sleep (either drug-induced or following sleep deprivation), since interictal epileptiform activity, particularly that associated with partial epilepsy, is often increased during drowsiness and light sleep. *In patients having frequent attacks, prolonged EEG with video-monitoring may allow the recording of an ictal event and confirm the*

Prolonged EEG with video-monitoring may allow the recording of an ictal event diagnosis. However, it should be noted that not all cortical spikes are recorded by scalp EEG, and hence an absence of ictal change in the EEG does not rule out the possibility of epilepsy. This is particularly the case for simple partial seizures, seizures arising in the mesial or orbital frontal regions, and seizures in which the only manifestation is a visceral aura.

6.8 How can the EEG help to clarify the seizure type?

The EEG in the generalized epilepsies typically shows the presence of generalized epileptiform discharges, often of the spike and wave variety, although polyspike activity is also not uncommon. ***Typical absence epilepsy (formerly known as "petit mal" epilepsy) is characterized by 3 per second spike and wave activity (Figure 22).*** Such activity can often be brought out during hyperventilation. In juvenile myoclonic epilepsy, photosensitivity (the development of epileptic activity in response to photic stimulation) is common (Figure 23), while the ictal and interictal EEG show generalized irregular spike and slow wave discharges. Slow spike and wave discharges may be seen in patients with Lennox-Gastaut syndrome (Figure 24).

Typical absence epilepsy can be characterized

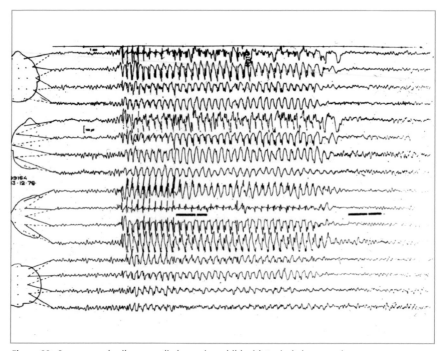

Figure 22. *3 per second spike wave discharge in a child with typical absence seizures (Courtesy of Dr Shelagh Smith).*

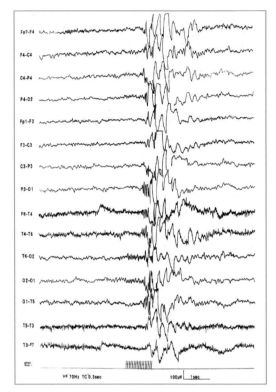

Figure 23. *Generalized spike wave discharge provoked by photic stimulation in case of idiopathic generalized epilepsy (Courtesy of Dr Shelagh Smith).*

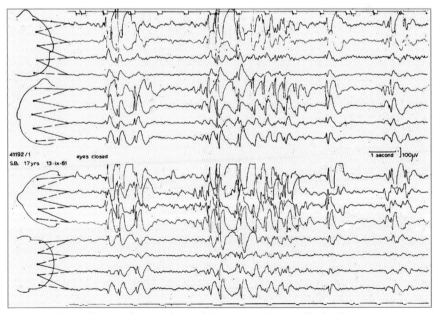

Figure 24. *Slow spike wave discharge (<2.5 Hz) in symptomatic generalized epilepsy (Courtesy of Dr Shelagh Smith).*

It is often difficult to distinguish idiopathic generalized seizures from secondarily generalized seizures on a clinical basis, particularly if the spread of seizure activity in the partial epilepsy occurs quickly so that no aura is experienced. ***An ictal EEG may demonstrate the partial onset of such seizures (Figure 25), while interictal EEGs may also raise this possibility by demonstrating focal epileptiform activity (Figure 26).*** However, caution is needed in the interpretation of the interictal EEG since both partial and generalized epileptic activity may occur in the same patient.

Ictal and interictal EEG issues

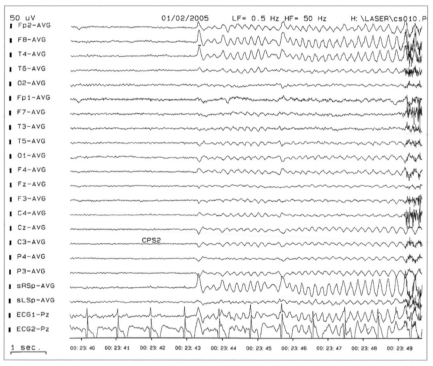

Figure 25. *Right temporal lobe seizure in unilateral hippocampal sclerosis (Courstesy of Dr Shelagh Smith).*

Apart from its use in identifying the seizure focus in some patients with symptomatic epilepsy (i.e. epilepsy secondary to a known cause), the EEG may also show typical features in idiopathic partial epilepsies such as benign epilepsy of childhood with centrotemporal spikes, and benign epilepsy of childhood with occipital paroxysms, rendering further investigation unnecessary in the presence of a classical clinical history.

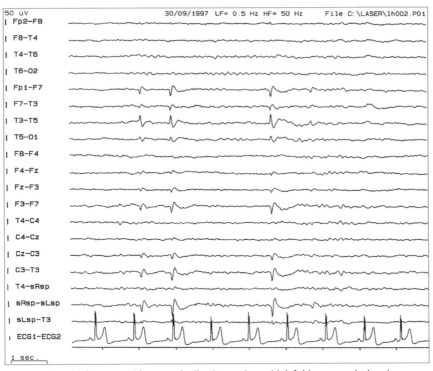

Figure 26. *Focal left antero-mid temporal spikes in a patient with left hippocampal sclerosis (Courtesy of Dr Shelagh Smith).*

6.9 Does prolonged EEG with video-monitoring have any role other than the diagnosis of epilepsy?

In addition to clarifying the diagnosis of epilepsy in some patients, prolonged EEG with video-monitoring plays a very important role in the evaluation of patients being considered for surgical treatment of their epilepsy. It allows close examination of the clinical features of the seizure, and the recording should include questioning of the patient during and after the seizure to assess responsiveness, verbal and memory function. Evaluation for post-ictal paresis should also be carried out. The clinical features may themselves permit accurate localization of the seizure discharge, with the EEG providing further information about the site of onset. *Caution is needed in the interpretation of both clinical and EEG features however, since false localization may occur.* Where doubt about the site of the epileptic focus remains after prolonged EEG with video-monitoring with scalp electrodes, recording with depth or subdural electrodes may be necessary.

> *Careful interpretation of clinical and EEG features*

6.10   Is an EEG indicated prior to discontinuation of medication?

There has been controversy as to whether interictal epileptiform activity is of prognostic significance with regard to recurrence of seizures in patients stopping antiepileptic medication. The available evidence suggests that in adults, the EEG is of limited help in predicting subsequent relapse. It may be of more use in patients with idiopathic generalized epilepsy. In children, an active interictal epileptiform disturbance probably indicates a slight increase in the risk of recurrent seizures.

Use of the EEG in predicting subsequent seizures

6.11   When should neuroimaging be performed?

In adults the chance of finding a structural lesion as a cause of seizures is greater than in children, and neuroimaging, preferably an MRI scan, should be performed in almost every case. (Where there are contraindications to MRI, or it is not available, a CT scan may be performed, but provides less information). Scanning is particularly important where the seizures are focal, where neurological abnormalities are found on examination, or where there is EEG evidence of a focal abnormality. Children with clinically obvious primary generalized epilepsy do not require neuroimaging, but a scan is warranted in most children with partial seizures except where these clearly conform to a "benign" syndrome such as benign epilepsy of childhood with centrotemporal spikes. Neuroimaging is justified in any child less than one year old presenting with epileptic seizures, since structural lesions are often present, most idiopathic epilepsies starting after this age.

Usefulness of the CT scan or MRI scan in adult diagnosis

6.12   What are the advantages of MRI scans over CT scans in people with epilepsy?

MRI scans have a number of advantages over CT scans. Certain abnormalities which may not be shown on CT scan because they are isodense with brain may be demonstrated by MRI scan: these include demyelinating lesions, encephalitis, and some low-grade gliomas. Neuronal migration disorders are one cause of seizures which may sometimes be apparent on CT scan but most often are only visualized by MRI. Mesial temporal sclerosis may also be demonstrated by MRI, and volumetric measurements can be used to demonstrate atrophy of the amygdala and hippocampus, which are often associated with temporal lobe epilepsy. Another advantage of magnetic resonance imaging is that it does not involve ionizing radiation, and is hence

Advantage of the MRI

thought not to constitute a biological hazard. Calcification (which may occur in oligodendrogliomas or cavernous angiomas) is better demonstrated by CT scanning. MRI also allows functional images of the brain and co-registration with EEG which may help locate epileptogenic sites.

Functional MRI (fMRI), which scans function rather than structure, is mainly a research tool. However, it has clinical applications in epilepsy particularly in pre-surgical evaluation (Figure 27 – fMRI- verbal memory activation). It is useful to determine laterality of speech function and memory and as such may eventually replace the Wada test (see section 8.4). Functional MRI also allows functional images of the brain and co-registration with EEG which may help locate epileptogenic sites (Figure 28 – simultaneous EEG-fMRI recording).

6.13 When are SPET and PET scanning indicated?

The main use of SPET (single photon emission tomography) and PET (positron emission tomography) in epilepsy is in pre-operative evaluation. PET provides better resolution than SPET

Pre-operative evaluation

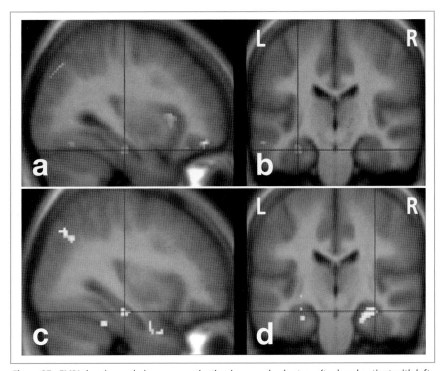

Figure 27. FMRI showing verbal memory activation in normal volunteers (top) and patient with left hippocampal sclerosis. (Courtesy of Professor John S. Duncan).

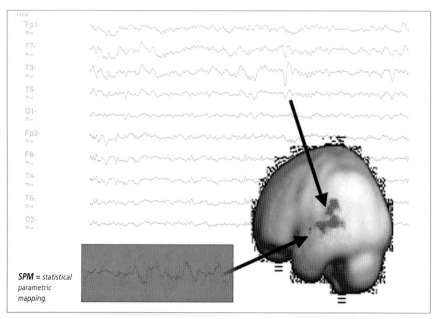

Figure 28. *Simultaneous EEG / fMRI - mapping of interictal epileptiform discharges. (Courtesy of Professor John S. Duncan)*

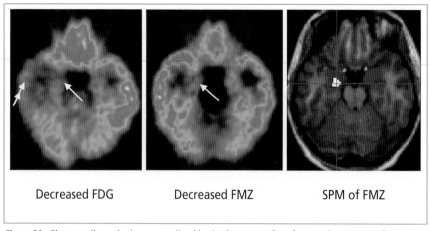

Decreased FDG   Decreased FMZ   SPM of FMZ

Figure 29. *Flumazenil uptake in a normalized brain. (courtesy of Professor John S. Duncan).*

scanning but requires a cyclotron on site since the isotopes used have very short half-lives. Interictally, unilaterally reduced cerebral glucose metabolism measured using 18-F-2-deoxyglucose (FDG) is seen in 70-80% of patients with complex partial seizures (Figure 29) usually over the temporal lobe. Ictal FDG-PET studies are rarely obtained, but may show increased glucose metabolism at the site of the epileptic focus. Cerebral blood flow may also be measured using ^{15}O labeled gases (by inhalation) or water (by injection) and give similar results to those obtained with FDG-PET, although the methods may not be as sensitive.

SPET scanning does not require an on-site cyclotron and is *less expensive then PET.* It provides similar information to that obtained for cerebral blood flow measurements with PET, but the resolution is not as good and the method is less sensitive (about 50% of patients with focal seizures having reduced interictal cerebral blood flow). However, in 15-20% of patients lateralization does not concur with the EEG results. The advantage of SPET over PET scanning is that ictal scans can be obtained because the half-lives of the isotopes are longer, increased blood flow being shown on the side of the EEG focus in 65-90% of patients.

SISCOM (Subtraction Ictal SPET co-registered to MRI) is a technique devised in an attempt to counteract the problems arising from the low resolution of SPET scanning. In this technique, the interictal and ictal SPET scans are electronically compared, one image being subtracted from the other and then superimposed on an MRI scan of the patient's brain. SISCOM allows accurate localization of the seizure focus in some cases of cryptogenic epilepsy.

6.14 When is neuropsychological testing appropriate?

People with epilepsy may be at risk of psychological problems for a variety of reasons. The epilepsy may produce problems of adjustment, and particularly in young children parental overprotection may impair social development. It is thought

The risk of psychological problems

that seizures themselves may cause brain damage if they are very prolonged or frequent. Subclinical epileptic discharges can cause transient cognitive defects and if the epilepsy is symptomatic, the underlying lesion may also be associated with problems of cognition. The adverse effect of antiepileptic drugs on mental functioning has become much more widely recognized in recent years. It could therefore be argued that neuropsychological assessment is appropriate in most people developing epilepsy. In practice, such assessment is not often performed and may not be readily available. Since, in the majority of people developing epilepsy, seizures are readily controlled with monotherapy using modern drugs, it would seem reasonable to reserve such assessment for people who have obvious or possible psychological or learning difficulties, and those whose seizures are intractable, particularly if surgery is contemplated.

CHAPTER 7

THE MEDICAL TREATMENT OF EPILEPSY

7.1   When should treatment for epilepsy be started?

The first requirement before antiepileptic medication is started is that the patient should have had a confirmed diagnosis of epileptic seizures. In practice this may be difficult, and it is not

Confirmed epileptic seizures before medication

uncommon for several months to elapse between the time of the first afebrile seizure and confirmation of the diagnosis of epilepsy.

The second issue of importance when considering treatment relates to the likelihood of recurrence after a first seizure. This has been estimated at between 27 and 84%. The differences between the results found by the various studies are largely methodological: in some, patients with a first seizure have been identified only at their first hospital visit, for example, so that patients having an early recurrence (before being seen) would be excluded, while in other studies, most people have received antiepileptic drugs after the initial seizure. Such factors are liable to reduce the apparent rate of recurrence.

The probability of a second seizure is greatest immediately after the initial event and falls thereafter. The etiology of the

Probability of a second seizure

seizures also influences the chance of recurrence: there is evidence that acute symptomatic seizures (those occurring in the context of an acute insult to the brain, such as stroke or encephalitis, or in association with metabolic derangement or drugs) are less likely to recur than idiopathic seizures or remote symptomatic seizures, while seizures occurring in patients with a neurological deficit present from birth have the highest rate of recurrence. There is controversy about the effect of age at onset of seizures on recurrence.

In Europe, most neurologists do not recommend starting antiepileptic treatment until the occurrence of a second seizure, unless there is a specific factor (such as the presence of a cerebral tumor, or the occurrence of unprovoked status epilepticus at presentation) which makes recurrence very likely. This reduces the chance of people taking antiepileptic drugs unnecessarily for long periods of time (the risk of a third seizure after a second has occurred is even greater than the risk of recurrence after a first seizure). This policy has recently been given support by the result of a large pragmatic clinical trial, the MESS study [1], which showed no difference in outcome in people who were treated after the first seizure and people who had the initiation of treatment deferred.

Specific factors examined

In the United States, it is often recommended that antiepileptic treatment is started after a first seizure. However, **the decision regarding when to start antiepileptic drugs must be discussed fully with the patient, and must take into account both medical and social considerations. If a patient expresses a strong wish to start treatment after a first seizure this should be taken into account.**

Medical and social considerations

Concern, first postulated by Gowers over 100 years ago that , "...the effect of a convulsion on the nerve centers is such as to render the occurrence of another more easy, to intensify the predisposition that already exists. Thus every fit may be said to be, in part, the result of those that have preceded it, the cause of those which follow it..." has not been supported by the MESS study and for the majority of patients antiepileptic treatment should only be considered after a second seizure.

A small number of patients have very infrequent seizures, perhaps one every few years. In these patients the need for treatment from the medical point of view is not great, and some patients prefer not to take medication every day in order to prevent a very occasional event. For others, however, the uncertainty as to when a seizure will occur or the wish to drive mean that they would prefer to take regular medication, and this is a reasonable choice.

Patient preference for treatment

A proportion of patients only experience seizures while asleep, and may prefer not to take medication. Other factors that should be considered when deciding whether antiepileptic treatment is appropriate include the type of epileptic seizure or syndrome, the likelihood of compliance with treatment, and the presumed etiology. The risk of sudden unexpected death in epilepsy (SUDEP) also needs to be considered. If a patient has seizures accompanied by a high risk of injury (such as atonic seizures) the need for treatment is greater than for patients with minor simple partial seizures having little effect on everyday life.

Some epilepsy syndromes, such as benign epilepsy of childhood with centrotemporal spikes, follow a benign course, and if seizures occur mainly during the night or are infrequent, medication may be unnecessary. Patients in whom seizures are regularly precipitated by alcohol (or its withdrawal) or abuse of drugs are better served by abstinence from the offending agent than by medication, with which they may not be compliant.

Compliance is of particular importance in the treatment of epilepsy, since withdrawal seizures may be precipitated by the abrupt cessation of medication. Some patients, such as those with malignant tumors or other progressive neurological conditions, are at higher risk of recurrence and in these patients, medication is usually appropriate after a single seizure.

Compliance is important

Patients whose seizures occur in the context of a metabolic disorder or acute insult to the brain, in contrast, are less likely to have a recurrence.

7.2 What advice should be given to patients starting treatment for epilepsy?

In some patients, ***seizures can be precipitated by certain stimuli.*** Examples of such precipitants include excessive alcohol intake, sleep deprivation, flickering lights (such as may occur with television screens, computer games and discotheques), and menstruation.

Avoidance of precipitants where feasible may be helpful, but most of these patients will nonetheless require medication to control unprovoked seizures. It should be stressed that only a few people with epilepsy are photosensitive, while the majority are able to enjoy discotheques and use computer screens without problem.

Unprovoked seizures

The need for medication to be taken regularly should be stressed, and the patient advised of the risk of withdrawal seizures if medication is abruptly withdrawn. The aims of treatment and the need for it to be continued even when seizures are controlled should be fully explained. Other issues that should be addressed include possible drug interactions (including the interaction of those drugs causing hepatic enzyme induction with the oral contraceptive pill).

The importance of medication

People often ask about the interaction of alcohol with antiepileptic drugs (AEDs). The majority of people are able to

Interaction with alcohol

take modest amounts of alcohol without a problem: they should be advised, however, that the sedative effects of some antiepileptic drugs may be enhanced.

7.3 What advice should be given to relatives and carers about the management of seizures?

Convulsive seizures may look frightening and advice should be given to relatives or carers as to how to cope with them. It should be stressed that the patient is not in pain and will usually have no recollection of the event afterwards, *seizures are generally self-limited, and serious injury is rare.* Attendance at hospital is seldom necessary.

Serious injury is rare

Patients should be made as comfortable as possible, preferably lying down (they should be eased to the floor if sitting), and the head should be cushioned. Any tight clothing or neckwear should be loosened. During seizures, patients should not be moved, unless they are in a dangerous place, for example in a road, by a fire or hot radiator, at the top of stairs or by the edge of water.

Do not open the patient's mouth

No attempt should be made to open the patient's mouth or force anything between the teeth. If the tongue is bitten during an attack, this almost invariably happens at the beginning, and well-meaning attempts to prevent it or protect the airway in this way usually result in damage. Broken teeth may be inhaled, causing secondary lung damage. When the seizure stops, the patient should be moved into the recovery position.

Partial attacks are usually less dramatic. During automatisms, patients may behave in a confused fashion and should generally be left undisturbed. Gentle restraint may be necessary if the automatism leads to dangerous wandering. Attempts at firm restraint, however, may increase agitation and confusion and provoke aggression.

No drinks or drugs following an attack... offer reassurance

No drinks should be given after an attack, nor should extra antiepileptic drugs be given. Onlookers are often worried that a patient may die during a seizure, but such an occurrence is exceedingly rare. *After a seizure*, it is important to *stay with the patient and offer reassurance* until the confused period has subsided and the patient has recovered fully.

If a seizure persists for more than 10 minutes, if a series of seizures occur, or if the seizure is particularly severe, then intravenous or rectal administration of diazepam is advisable (assuming facilities are available). Buccal midazolam is an alternative, although this is an unlicensed indication.

7.4   How should drug treatment be instituted?

Approximately 60-70% of patients developing epilepsy will have their seizures controlled with monotherapy using a first-line drug and research has shown that in most patients, seizure control is optimal with monotherapy, while adverse effects are minimized. Drug interactions and poor compliance are also more likely with polytherapy. However, 10-15% of patients require two drugs for optimal seizure control.

The patient should be treated initially with a first-line drug appropriate to the seizure-type. The drug is usually started at a low dose, which is gradually increased until either the seizures are controlled, or the patient experiences side effects.

Initial treatment with first-line drug

Some drugs are particularly liable to cause toxic symptoms if the dose is increased too quickly, and every effort should be made to avoid this situation, since it may well make the patient reluctant to continue medication. If the first-line drug fails to control seizures or is not tolerated, another first-line drug is tried and the previous drug withdrawn.

7.5   What is the drug of choice in patients with generalized tonic clonic seizures?

Carbamazepine, lamotrigine, levetiracetam, oxcarbazepine, sodium valproate and topiramate are all effective in the treatment of generalized tonic clonic seizures, whether primary or secondarily generalized. Sodium valproate has traditionally

Effective drugs in tonic-clonic seizures

been used as first line drug for generalized seizures and carbamazepine for partial onset seizures. However, the SANAD study [2,3] suggests that while sodium valproate is still the drug of choice for generalized seizures, lamotrigine may be better tolerated than, and as effective as, carbamazepine in the treatment of partial onset seizures. In women with generalized epilepsy lamotrigine may be preferred to valproate in view of the risk of teratogenicity with the latter: levetiracetam may also prove to be an option but further information on its teratogenic potential is required before it can be recommended in pregnancy.

7.6 Which other drugs are helpful in the treatment of generalized epileptic seizures?

In patients with *true absence attacks alone, ethosuximide is also an effective drug and is an alternative to sodium valproate.* Levetiracetam and benzodiazepines (such as clonazepam) may be helpful in the treatment of myoclonus.

True absence attacks

7.7 Which drugs may be used in the treatment of partial seizures?

Carbamazepine, lamotrigine, levetiracetam, oxcarbazepine, sodium valproate and topiramate are effective options in this respect. *Clobazam, gabapentin, pregabalin, tiagabine, and zonisamide may all be helpful in the management of partial seizures as second line drugs.* Some of these are newer drugs and are as yet only marketed for the treatment of refractory seizures in certain countries.

Medication for partial seizures

7.8 What is the procedure if the first drug fails?

If treatment with a drug appropriate for the seizure type fails in any patient with a new diagnosis of epilepsy, the patient should be reassessed, with particular attention to whether the diagnosis of epilepsy is still correct, and whether the seizures have an underlying etiology which remains to be identified. Enquiries should also be made about compliance with medication, and serum drug levels checked if feasible. Assuming these are satisfactory, another appropriate drug should be commenced, and the initial drug gradually withdrawn.

Reassess the diagnosis

Check compliance and drug levels

The dose of the second drug should be titrated in the same manner as the first until seizures are controlled or adverse effects occur. If the second drug also fails in monotherapy, a combination of two drugs appropriate to the seizure type may be tried.

If the seizures remain uncontrolled, attention should again be directed to the diagnosis of epilepsy and underlying etiology of the seizures. One of the first-line drugs (whichever is least well-tolerated) should then be gradually replaced by a second-line drug; if the latter is effective, subsequent gradual withdrawal of the initial drug can be considered. Other second-line drugs may be tried in turn if the seizures remain

Consider second-line drugs

intractable, and the use of experimental antiepileptic agents considered, preferably as part of a controlled trial.

7.9 What problems are encountered when antiepileptic drugs are used in patients with renal or hepatic disease?

Sodium valproate is contraindicated in patients with active liver disease, in whom it may cause acute hepatic failure. Other antiepileptic drugs that are metabolised in the liver include carbamazepine, phenytoin, phenobarbital, ethosuximide, lamotrigine, the benzodiazepines, and paraldehyde. These drugs should be used with caution in patients with hepatic impairment.

Metabolism in the liver and kidney

Drugs which are excreted via the kidney, at least in part, or which have active metabolites which are excreted in the urine include ethosuximide, phenobarbital, the benzodiazepines, lamotrigine, levetiracetam and gabapentin, and care should be taken if these drugs are given to patients with renal impairment. Acetazolamide should be avoided if renal impairment is severe.

7.10 What precautions should be taken when prescribing antiepileptic drugs for the elderly?

A special effort should be made to avoid polytherapy in the elderly, both because of the risk of drug interactions and the difficulties which may be encountered in coping with a complicated regime.

Drug interaction in the elderly

Compliance may be improved if instructions for taking the drugs are written down. There is an increased susceptibility to certain drugs, particularly those which may cause sedation, in old age, and such drugs should be used with care. It should also be remembered that many elderly people have a degree of renal impairment.

7.11 When should antiepileptic drug levels be monitored?

The dose of drugs required by each patient depends largely on the clinical response. In general, if a patient fails to respond to a small dose of an appropriate drug, the dose should be gradually increased until either the seizures are controlled, or evidence of toxicity or other adverse effects occur. However, situations in which drug-level monitoring may be helpful are shown in Table 6.

Clinical response to dosages

Monitoring of serum drug levels is most helpful in the case of phenytoin, because of its non-linear kinetics. Monitoring of carbamazepine, phenobarbital, ethosuximide, gabapentin, lamotrigine, tiagabine, topiramate, levetiracetam, pregabalin and zonisamide levels is less helpful but may sometimes be useful in selected patients.

Monitoring serum drug levels

7.12 What factors determine the likelihood of achieving seizure control?

The likelihood of achieving seizure control is determined in part by the epilepsy syndrome and seizure type. Many of the idiopathic epilepsies have a good prognosis. Primary generalized epilepsy is usually amenable to treatment with sodium valproate provided that the drug is well tolerated. However, some syndromes, such as juvenile myoclonic epilepsy, may require long-term treatment.

Good prognosis for idiopathic epilepsies

The seizures of benign epilepsy of childhood with centrotemporal spikes almost invariably remit during the second decade, and may not require treatment at all if infrequent. Benign epilepsy of childhood with occipital paroxysms also has an excellent prognosis. In contrast, other syndromes such as West syndrome and Lennox-Gastaut syndrome imply a poor prognosis, both for seizure type and for intellectual development.

7.13 What are the adverse effects of medication?

The adverse effects of AEDs fall into four groups: acute dose-related effects (intoxication), chronic toxic effects, idiosyncratic (allergic) effects and teratogenicity. *Acute dose-related effects*

Effects of medication

- To check compliance in patients with refractory seizures
- To guide dosage when using drugs with difficult pharmacokinetics eg., phenytoin
- To guide dosage when using polytherapy, in patients with renal or hepatic disease, and in patients in whom toxicity is difficult to assess (eg, those with learning difficulties)
- To guide dosage in pregnant patients
- Controlled trials of antiepileptic drugs
- To document drug toxicity and interactions

Table 6. *Indications for monitoring of serum drug levels.*

are similar for all the antiepileptic drugs, though they differ in degree: they include dizziness, ataxia, nystagmus, nausea, visual disturbances, headaches and drowsiness.

The chronic toxic effects of AEDs tend to be more subtle, often developing insidiously. They may affect many systems, producing neurological, hematological, hepatic, immunological, metabolic, endocrine, connective tissue, gastrointestinal and other changes, although such changes are often of little clinical significance. The most important of the chronic toxic effects are usually neurological, including sedation, lethargy, mental slowing, memory disturbance, depression, irritability and aggression.

Idiosyncratic adverse effects usually develop soon after the initiation of the treatment, and may be potentially serious. The drugs should be withdrawn if they occur. The most common is skin rash, which is occasionally severe, such as Stevens-Johnson syndrome or exfoliative dermatitis, but usually mild. Other serious but

Idiosyncratic effects

rare idiosyncratic effects are agranulocytosis or pancytopenia (described with phenytoin, carbamazepine, levetiracetam and felbamate), pancreatitis and acute hepatic failure (reported with phenytoin, valproate, felbamate, levetiracetam and lamotrigine).

Generalized lymphadenopathy and a lupus-like syndrome may also occur as allergic phenomena. Teratogenicity is discussed further in Chapter 9.

7.14 What help can be given to patients in whom medical management is unsuccessful?

As soon as it becomes clear that the seizures will not be easily controlled by medical means, and while second-line drugs are still being tried, consideration should be given to the suitability of the patient for epilepsy surgery (see Chapter 8). Appropriate investigations should be undertaken (including MRI if not already performed, and EEG monitoring to localize the site of seizure onset). *Epilepsy*

Specialist centers for surgery

surgery is best carried out in a specialist center and contact should be made with one at an early stage, since many specialists involved with epilepsy surgery prefer to carry out investigations themselves.

7.15 When and how should antiepileptic treatment be withdrawn?

The decision as to when to withdraw antiepileptic treatment is always difficult, particularly in adults in whom considerations such as driving and employment may be affected by a recurrence of seizures. The patient should be counselled about the risk of relapse and its possible consequences before any reduction in dose is undertaken. *It is usually advised that patients should have been seizure-free for at least two years, and preferably longer, before drug withdrawal is attempted. In some countries it is advised that the patient should stop driving during drug withdrawal and for a defined period afterwards.*

Withdrawal of drug treatment

Drugs should be withdrawn slowly over a period of several months. If the patient is taking polytherapy, withdrawal of one drug should be completed before reduction of the dose of the other drug is undertaken.

7.16 What is the risk of recurrence of seizures after stopping medication? What factors influence this?

Most studies suggest that the risk of recurrence of seizures after two years of seizure freedom following withdrawal of antiepileptic medication is about 20% in children and 40% in adults. *Factors influencing the likelihood of relapse include the duration of epilepsy prior to seizure control* (the prognosis being worse in those whose seizures were initially difficult to control), *the duration of remission* (the prognosis being better in those with long remission prior to drug withdrawal), *seizure type* (idiopathic epilepsy, except juvenile myoclonic epilepsy, usually having a better prognosis than symptomatic epilepsy), and *the presence of additional handicaps.*

Factors influencing relapse

The influence of the EEG on prognosis following drug withdrawal is controversial, some studies suggesting a relationship between the presence of epileptic abnormalities and the likelihood of relapse, while others do not confirm this. The association appears to be greater in children than adults.

The majority of *patients who relapse following drug withdrawal do so within one year.* If treatment is reinstated, seizure control is usually regained, but difficulties may be experienced in approximately 15% of patients.

Timescale for relapse

7.17 Is there any treatment for epilepsy which does not require the use of drugs?

Not all people with epilepsy require treatment with antiepileptic drugs, either because they have very mild or infrequent seizures. *Although the majority of people with more severe epilepsy will require drug therapy, there may be other means by which their seizure control can be improved.*

Controlling severe epilepsy

The avoidance of factors known to precipitate seizures has already been discussed. Other non-pharmacological methods for averting seizures depend on specific maneuvers undertaken at the onset of an aura, to prevent progression of the seizure. Some people find that they may achieve this by intense concentration, others by relaxation. It may be helpful to teach patients breathing exercises to prevent hyperventilation, with its accompanying risk of facilitation of seizures, in these circumstances. Other techniques which may be helpful include intense motor activity or sensory stimulation.

A few children with intractable seizures, particularly in the context of Lennox-Gastaut syndrome and myoclonic-astatic epilepsy, may benefit from a high-fat diet, the so-called ketogenic diet. This diet is not useful in adults with epilepsy.

Vagal nerve stimulation is a recent, palliative development in the treatment of epilepsy. It involves the long-term placement of an electrode to stimulate the vagal nerve, either continuously or on demand. It has been reported to be effective in a small proportion of patients with chronic partial epilepsy, although the chance of patients becoming seizure-free is low.

Vagal nerve stimulation

7.18 How should status epilepticus be treated?

Status epilepticus is a neurological emergency, since the longer it is allowed to continue, the greater the risk of permanent cerebral damage, and the harder it becomes to control.

Risk of cerebral damage

Efforts should be directed at ensuring the adequacy of cardiorespiratory function, controlling the clinical and electrical manifestations of seizure activity, treating the underlying cause and correcting metabolic imbalance occurring as a result of the status.

On the patient's arrival in hospital, an airway should be inserted and oxygen given. An intravenous cannula should be inserted, and blood taken for urea and electrolytes, blood glucose, serum calcium and magnesium, anticonvulsant levels (if a patient is known to have epilepsy), and full blood count. Arterial blood gases should be measured if clinically appropriate. Intravenous lorazepam or diazepam (the usual dose in adults being lorazepam 4mg or diazepam 10-20mg) should be administered by slow injection, care being taken to observe for any evidence of respiratory depression.

Oxygen and blood tests

Monitor the heart and blood pressure

In most patients, seizure activity will cease with this treatment. However, there is a risk of recurrence of seizures as the serum level of the benzodiazepine drops, and a loading dose of phenytoin should therefore also be administered, the total dose being 15mg/kg at a rate of less than 50mg per minute. Cardiac monitoring should be carried out during the injection, and the blood pressure checked. In patients in whom status is due to antiepileptic drug withdrawal, the patient's usual medication should be re-established as soon as possible.

Persistent seizure activity

In patients in whom seizure activity persists despite the initial dose of phenytoin, a further slow injection of phenytoin (5mg/kg) should be given, repeated if necessary until a total of phenytoin 30mg/kg has been administered. These patients are also likely to be developing secondary metabolic disturbances as a result of the status, including electrolyte imbalance, hypoglycemia, dehydration, hyperpyrexia and lactic acidosis.

Secondary disturbances

The acidosis, if mild, is likely to correct itself: the other abnormalities should be actively treated. Arterial blood gases should be measured, if not already done.

Intravenous phenobarbital is another option. As it may cause respiratory depression, close monitoring is mandatory, so that the patient can be intubated and mechanically ventilated if necessary.

EEG monitoring

In patients in whom all other measures fail, elective ventilation in association with thiopentone infusion may be necessary. In this instance, EEG monitoring is necessary to ensure that suppression of seizure activity is complete. EEG monitoring is also important to exclude the possibility of pseudostatus epilepticus, which is common, particularly in patients referred to tertiary centers for further treatment.

7.19 Which antiepileptic drugs are currently available?

This section provides a general overview of all available AEDs. We have tried to ensure that all drug related information here provided is accurate but such information may change from time to time and clinicians are strongly advised to consult manufacturers' information sheets and national prescribing guidelines where available before prescribing drugs. In some cases, recommendations may be outside licensed indications.

The following antiepileptic drugs are currently available:

Acetazolamide	Ethosuximide	Oxcarbazepine	Stiripentol
ACTH	Felbamate	Paraldehyde	Sulthiame
Carbamazepine	Gabapentin	Phenobarbital	Tiagabine
Chlormethiazole	Lamotrigine	Phenytoin	Topiramate
Clobazam	Levetiracetam	Piracetam	Valproate
Clonazepam	Lorazepam	Pregabalin	Vigabatrin
Diazepam	Nitrazepam	Primidone	Zonisamide

ACETAZOLAMIDE

Acetazolamide is a carbonic anhydrase inhibitor which is still used occasionally as an antiepileptic drug in the treatment of generalized tonic clonic, absence and complex partial seizures. Its main current use is in the treatment of glaucoma.

Acetazolamide's major drawback is that, in many patients who initially derive benefit from the drug, tolerance develops, usually after several months, and seizure control is lost. Acetazolamide is available in tablet form and as an infusion for intravenous use. The usual daily maintenance dose is 250 -1000mg. Adverse effects include nausea, diarrhea, taste disturbance, loss of appetite, paraesthesias, arthralgia, headache, dizziness, fatigue, irritability, depression, thirst, polyuria, metabolic acidosis, drowsiness, confusion, and hearing disturbances. Renal stones may also occur. Blood dyscrasias and Stevens-Johnson syndrome have also been reported albeit very rarely. Teratogenicity has been noted in animals but there are no human data on this.

ADRENOCORTICOTROPHIC HORMONE (ACTH)

This corticosteroid is useful in the treatment of infantile spasms
(West syndrome) although there is no universal agreement about its use.
It is given by intramuscular injection, usually in reducing doses over a period
of three months. Adverse effects of the drug include leukocytosis, irritability,
hypertension, vomiting, peripheral edema, Cushingoid facies, gastrointestinal
hemorrhage, electrolyte disturbances, reversible cerebral atrophy, sepsis,
hyperglycemia, and congestive heart failure.

CARBAMAZEPINE

Carbamazepine is a tricyclic derivative used in the treatment of epilepsy since
the 1960s, and is still one of the first-line drugs in the treatment of all types of
partial seizures and generalized tonic clonic seizures. It is, however, not a broad
spectrum drug and may exacerbate generalized seizures particularly absence
and myoclonic seizures.

Carbamazepine is available in tablet form, suppositories, and liquid, but not as
an injectable preparation. The usual daily dose of carbamazepine in adults is
400-1600mg. It is a potent auto-inducer, and must be started at a low dose
(100-200mg in an adult) to keep development of transient neurotoxicity at a
minimum. Indeed, toxic symptoms are common if the dose of the drug is
increased too quickly, and may also occur during long term administration as a
time-locked phenomenon after each dose particularly if the conventional
formulation is used. Controlled release preparations are, therefore, preferable
as they reduce toxicity associated with these peak plasma concentrations of the
drug and are also suitable for twice daily administration.

The most common unwanted effect of carbamazepine is skin rash, which occurs
in up to 5-6% of patients and may be serious in up to 10% of these. Other
adverse effects include nausea, diplopia, nystagmus, dizziness, fatigue and
headache. Other common side effects include drowsiness, ataxia, confusion
and agitation (particularly in the elderly), hyponatremia, and neutropenia. The
neutropenia does not usually cause any clinical manifestations. Hyponatremia
seen with carbamazepine is rarely symptomatic but occasionally leads to
confusion, peripheral edema, and an increase in the number of seizures. Very
rare side effects include hepatitis, Stevens-Johnson syndrome, toxic epidermal
necrolysis, and cardiac conduction disturbances. Fluid retention may limit the

use of carbamazepine in the elderly or those with cardiac failure. In addition, it may aggravate bradycardia in patients with heart disease. Although some congenital malformations have been reported in children exposed to carbamazepine in utero, overall this drug is felt to be relatively safe during pregnancy.

Carbamazepine, as an enzyme inducer, reduces the effectiveness of several drugs, such as oral contraceptives, steroids, haloperidol, theophylline, and warfarin. Conversely, other drugs inhibit its metabolism which may result in neurotoxicity; these include cimetidine, danazol, dextropropoxyphene, diltiazem, erythromycin, isoniazid, verapamil, and viloxazine. Interactions of carbamazepine with other antiepileptic drugs are also common. Carbamazepine increases the clearance particularly of ethosuximide, sodium valproate, topiramate and lamotrigine. Inhibition or enzyme induction is seen with phenobarbital, phenytoin, or primidone with usually small but unpredictable changes in the plasma concentrations of these drugs.

CHLORMETHIAZOLE

Chlormethiazole is available as an intravenous preparation for infusion in the treatment of status epilepticus. There is, however, little evidence to support its use for this indication. Adverse effects include respiratory depression, tachycardia, hypotension, depressed conscious level, hyponatraemia, nasal congestion and headache.

CLOBAZAM

Clobazam is a 1,5 benzodiazepine used as a second-line drug and effective against all seizure types. It is given orally, the usual dose being 10-30mg at night to avoid daytime drowsiness and sedation.

As with other benzodiazepines, tolerance occurs frequently, and over 50% of patients who initially have an excellent response will revert to their previous state within six months. In some patients however, it remains useful in the long term; at present there is no way of predicting who will develop tolerance and who will not. Clobazam is very useful as a drug for intermittent use. As such it can be helpful in the management of catamenial epilepsy and taken as required in patients in whom seizures occur in clusters. Clobazam can also be used to prevent seizures in the short term, for example to cover patients for such special events as holidays, weddings, family gatherings and so on. It can also be used to provide cover to patients at the time of withdrawal of other drugs.

The most common side effect of clobazam apart from sedation, is ataxia and this generally decreases on continued use. Less frequent adverse effects include vertigo, headache, confusion, depression, slurred speech, tremor, visual disturbances, irritability, urinary retention, changes in salivation, and amnesia. It has little potential for interactions. Its teratogenic profile is unknown in women with epilepsy and its use is not recommended during pregnancy particularly in the first trimester.

CLONAZEPAM

Clonazepam is particularly helpful in the treatment of myoclonus and photosensitive seizures, although it may also be beneficial as a second-line drug in most other seizure types. As with other benzodiazepines, tolerance to its initial antiepileptic action is a disadvantage although this is less common than with clobazam. Tolerance may develop in up to 30% of patients in whom the drug was initially beneficial. The starting dose of clonazepam is usually 0.5mg, increasing if necessary to a total dose of up to 6-8mg daily. Clonazepam is available as an intravenous preparation for infusion in the treatment of status epilepticus although lorazepam is a better drug for this indication. Sedation is more common than with clobazam, occurring initially in up to 50% of patients, although this symptom often improves with time. Other adverse effects include ataxia, muscle weakness, behavioral problems, nausea, hypersalivation, weight gain, and rarely, hematological effects. The drug should be withdrawn slowly to avoid the risk of withdrawal seizures. It is not recommended for use during pregnancy.

DIAZEPAM

This drug is used in the management of serial seizures and status epilepticus. There is no place for it in the maintenance treatment of epilepsy. It is usually given intravenously in the treatment of status epilepticus, the typical dose in adults being 10-20mg. Its use in this situation has to some extent been superseded by the use of intravenous lorazepam.

Seizures may recur as the plasma level falls, and therefore the administration of additional medication (such as intravenous phenytoin) is advisable. Diazepam is also rapidly absorbed rectally and this is a useful route of administration in the treatment of serial or prolonged seizures, allowing administration by parents or other carers and potentially avoiding the need for hospital admission. Adverse effects include sedation, respiratory depression, hypotension, drowsiness, vertigo, ataxia, blurred vision and amnesia.

ETHOSUXIMIDE

The only use of ethosuximide is in the treatment of typical absence seizures: where these co-exist with other seizure types, valproate is usually the first treatment of choice. Ethosuximide is available in tablet form and syrup. The typical daily maintenance dose of this drug is between 500-1000mg. Adverse effects include nausea and vomiting, headaches, anorexia, abdominal discomfort, sedation, movement disorders and skin rash. Very rarely it can cause psychotic episodes with paranoid ideation, aplastic anemia, systemic lupus erythematosus, and Stevens-Johnson syndrome. Ethosuximide-induced headache and abdominal pain can be severe in some patients.

Ethosuximide does not inhibit or induce the metabolism of other drugs but its clearance is reduced by valproate and toxicity may occur if these drugs are used together. Despite the fact that this drug has been available for many years, there is not enough data on its potential teratogenicity in humans and it should be used cautiously during pregnancy.

FELBAMATE

Felbamate is an effective broad spectrum drug useful particularly in refractory partial epilepsy: it was the first antiepileptic drug to have shown some efficacy as add-on treatment in refractory Lennox-Gastaut syndrome. It is available as tablets and oral solution. The usual dose is between 1800 and 4800mg/day. Its use is currently restricted to very refractory cases for safety reasons as it has been associated with an idiosyncratic reaction leading to aplastic anemia or hepatotoxicity. These rare but often fatal reactions may affect about 1 in 4,000 people exposed. Felbamate is licensed for use as a "last resort" drug in many countries. In view of its safety profile it seems prudent to limit its use to specialist centers in severe intractable cases. It is currently not licensed in the United Kingdom but can be obtained for selected cases on a named-patient basis. It interacts with many drugs and this needs to be taken into consideration when using felbamate. With regard to antiepileptic drugs, felbamate exhibits significant interactions with phenytoin, carbamazepine and valproic acid. It should be avoided during pregnancy.

FOSPHENYTOIN

Fosphenytoin, a pro-drug of phenytoin (see below), is a preparation for infusion that can be administered intravenously more rapidly than phenytoin and causes fewer injection site reactions than phenytoin. It has no other major advantages over phenytoin. Its only indication is as an alternative to phenytoin in the treatment of status epilepticus.

GABAPENTIN

Gabapentin, an amino acid, is a mild antiepileptic drug occasionally useful as add-on treatment of partial seizures. It is not effective for any other seizure type and it may exacerbate generalized seizures particularly myoclonic jerks. Its major indication currently is as an analgesic for chronic neuropathic pain. It is only available in tablet form. The typical daily maintenance dose of this drug for epilepsy is 2,400-4,800mg. Side effects of gabapentin include nausea, vomiting, peripheral edema, dizziness, drowsiness, ataxia, tremor, asthenia, emotional lability, weight gain, dysarthria, and diplopia. Rare side effects include pancreatitis, depression, psychosis, headache, myalgia, and urinary incontinence, hepatitis, jaundice, movement disorders, thrombocytopenia, and acute renal failure. Gabapentin is devoid of interactions and this is one of the few advantages of this drug. Not enough human exposure data has been accumulated to give it a clear bill of health with regard to teratogenicity and it should be used cautiously in women of child bearing potential.

LAMOTRIGINE

Lamotrigine was originally developed for its antifolate activity following suggestions of a relationship between folate and epilepsy. Its mode of action, however, is not related to its weak antifolate property and is thought to be due mainly to its potential to modulate sodium channels. It is a first line drug for partial and generalized seizures and as such a broad spectrum drug. It may, however, occasionally exacerbate myoclonic seizures particularly as part of Severe Myoclonic Epilepsy of infancy. Lamotrigine is only available as tablets and dispersible tablets. Its usual maintenance dose in monotherapy is between 100-400mg/day. The initiation of lamotrigine therapy should be at a very low dose with a slow upward titration to decrease the risk of the development of skin rash, which is an important side effect. The rash may be severe and lead to Stevens-Johnson syndrome in some rare cases, particularly if the medication is not stopped promptly. Other side effects include nausea, fatigue, dizziness, insomnia, tremor, agitation, confusion, hallucinations, and blood disorders (including leucopenia, thrombocytopenia, pancytopenia). Lamotrigine has the potential for interaction. The elimination of lamotrigine is accelerated by enzyme-inducing antiepileptic drugs, such as carbamazepine, phenytoin, and phenobarbital, and inhibited by valproate. Therefore, if lamotrigine is used as an add-on, the dose and titration schedule need to be adjusted according to the concomitant medication. In addition, in women, lamotrigine levels may be reduced, occasionally dramatically, by the addition of the combined oral contraceptive pill or during pregnancy, and dose adjustments may be necessary to avoid breakthrough seizures. Lamotrigine seems to be relatively safe with regard to teratogenicity particularly if low doses are used.

LEVETIRACETAM

Levetiracetam, an analogue of the anti-myoclonic drug piracetam (see below), is a broad spectrum antiepileptic drug. Its exact mode of action is unknown but it is thought to be related to its strong binding to the SV2A receptor. It is effective against partial and generalized seizures including those associated with juvenile myoclonic epilepsy. It may be used as a first line treatment or as an add-on. It is available in tablet form, oral solution and as a preparation for infusion for patients temporarily unable to take the drug orally or who require prompt antiepileptic drug loading.

The usual maintenance dose of levetiracetam for adults ranges from 750 to 3,000mg/day. It is generally well tolerated. The most frequent side effects encountered in clinical practice are lethargy, irritability, ataxia, nausea and vomiting, drowsiness, dizziness, headache, tremor, hyperkinesia, emotional lability, irritability, insomnia, anxiety, anorexia, and diplopia. Rare side effects include confusion, psychosis, leucopenia, thrombocytopenia and alopecia. Post-marketing experience has shown rare side effects include hepatitis and pancreatitis. Like other antiepileptic drugs levetiracetam should be started at a low dose and titrated up weekly to initial target dose. However, if there are clinical needs and under supervision, levetiracetam can be started at the maintenance dose either orally or as intravenous infusion. No clinically relevant interactions with other drugs have yet been described, as the drug is excreted mostly unchanged. However, it may have pharmacodynamic interactions with other antiepileptic drugs particularly carbamazepine. Not enough human exposure data has been accumulated to give it a clear bill of health with regard to teratogenicity.

LORAZEPAM

The benzodiazepine, lorazepam, given intravenously, controls seizures in a great number of patients with status epilepticus, for which it is a first-line drug. There is no place for it in the maintenance treatment of epilepsy. In adults, it is given in a dose of 4mg over two minutes, repeated if necessary after 15 minutes. Adverse effects include sedation, amnesia, dysarthria, delirium, hallucinations, and respiratory depression.

MIDAZOLAM

This short acting benzodiazepine is licensed for anesthesia, sedation and for the short term treatment of insomnia. It is, however, increasingly being used off licence buccally or nasally as a rescue medication for serial seizures and prolonged seizures in preference to rectal diazepam.

NITRAZEPAM

Nitrazepam, a potent benzodiazepine, is occasionally used in the treatment of infantile spasms. Like other benzodiazepines, tolerance may occur. In addition, it is very sedative and this limits its use.

PARALDEHYDE

This drug may occasionally be helpful in the treatment of serial seizures and status epilepticus although it is not currently generally available.

PHENOBARBITAL

Phenobarbital is an effective broad spectrum antiepileptic drug effective against most seizures types, intravenously or in chronic oral use. Currently, it is hardly used in developed countries as a chronic oral use drug, although it is used in emergency situations intravenously. In patients controlled at low daily doses, phenobarbital is a relatively cost-effective and well tolerated medication and is used especially in resource poor countries. The mode of action of phenobarbital

is probably mediated by the GABA receptor, though it is not clearly defined. The main disadvantages of phenobarbital are its potential to affect cognition, and pharmacokinetic interactions. It is available as tablets, oral solution and as an infusion. The usual maintenance dose is between 30 and 120 mg/day. Common side effects are drowsiness, depression, lethargy, cognitive slowing, Dupuytren's contracture, ataxia and allergic skin reactions. In the elderly, hyperactivity, restlessness and confusion may be seen, while hyperkinesia is a problem in children. Megaloblastic anemia is a chronic side effect and the use of concomitant folic acid supplementation is recommended. Phenobarbital interacts with a number of drugs, antiepileptic or otherwise, and this must be taken into account when using it: it interacts with steroids, antibiotics, oral contraceptives and other drugs. It decreases the levels of carbamazepine, lamotrigine, phenytoin, valproate, zonisamide and ethosuximide.
It is potentially teratogenic and its use during pregnancy should be avoided if possible.

PHENYTOIN

Phenytoin is an effective oral treatment for partial and tonic-clonic seizures, and is also useful intravenously in status epilepticus. However, because of its great potential to cause chronic side effects and pharmacokinetic interactions, it is now not used as first-line therapy in many countries. Phenytoin is available as capsules, tablets, suspension and injection. There may be differences in bioavailability between different oral preparations and patients stabilized on one formulation should continue to receive the same formulation.

The usual daily dose, which may be given as a single dose, is 200-400mg. Intravenous phenytoin is useful in patients unable to take the drug by the gastrointestinal route, and those with serial seizures or in status epilepticus. Since it may cause heart block if infused too quickly it should be administered with caution and at a rate not exceeding 50mg/minute. It should never be given intramuscularly, since absorption by this route is slow and unreliable, and tissue necrosis may occur.

The commonest side effects include cosmetic changes such as gingival hyperplasia, acne, hirsutism, facial coarsening and neuropsychiatric disturbance particularly depression, fatigue, and cognitive slowing. Other side effects include nausea, tremor, paraesthesias, dizziness, headache, anorexia and skin rash. Rarely, it may cause hepatoxicity, peripheral neuropathy, Dupuytren's contracture, lymphadenopathy, osteomalacia, megaloblastic anemia, leucopenia, thrombocytopenia, lupus erythematosus, and Stevens-Johnson syndrome. The use of concomitant folic acid supplementation with phenytoin is recommended. It has nonlinear pharmacokinetics and this can result in large increases in plasma concentrations even with small dose increments; conversely, levels may fall abruptly even with modest dose reduction. Routine monitoring of plasma levels of phenytoin is recommended. Phenytoin is a potent enzyme inducer, and as such can be expected to cause interactions with other drugs such as antiepileptic drugs, anticoagulants, steroids, cyclosporin, and oral contraceptives. Conversely, the metabolism of phenytoin can be inhibited by enzyme inducers such as allopurinol, chloramphenicol, cimetidine, isoniazid, metronidazol, phenothiazines, and sulphonamides. Its use should, if possible, be avoided during pregnancy.

PREGABALIN

Pregabalin, an analogue of GABA, and closely related to gabapentin, selectively binds to a subunit of voltage-gated calcium channels and this seems to be responsible for its antiepileptic action although the exact mode is unknown. It is a second line antiepileptic for partial seizures. It is unlikely to be of help in generalized seizures and there are concerns that it could exacerbate some forms of seizures, particularly myoclonic and absence seizures. In addition to its antiepileptic action, pregabalin is also used as an analgesic and in general anxiety disorders. The usual maintenance dose for adults with epilepsy ranges from 150 to 600 mg/day. Pregabalin is only available as capsules.

Its side effects include dizziness, drowsiness, irritability, speech disorder, paraesthesias, confusion, fatigue, weight gain and visual disturbances. Less common side effects include increased salivation, taste disturbance, edema, nasal dryness, stupor, depression, insomnia, mood swings, asthenia, muscle cramp, and rash. Rare effects include pancreatitis, arrhythmia, rhinitis, menstrual disturbances, breast discharge, breast hypertrophy, neutropenia, rhabdomyolysis, and renal failure. Like gabapentin, it seems devoid of any clinically significant interactions. Not enough human exposure data has been accumulated to give it a clear bill of health with regard to teratogenicity.

PIRACETAM

Piracetam is a pyrrolidine acetamate that has been used as a memory "enhancer" in some European countries for a number of years; it has, however, never been shown to be effective. Piracetam is, nevertheless, a very effective anti-myoclonic drug. The mode of action of this drug is unknown.

Piracetam is available in tablets and also as oral solution. The usual daily dose ranges from 7200mg to 20,000mg. There are no known drug interactions and it has relatively few side effects. Diarrhea, weight gain, insomnia, depression and hyperkinesias have been associated with it, particularly in high doses. Its use should be avoided during pregnancy.

PRIMIDONE

Primidone is a barbiturate that is largely metabolized to phenobarbital, and its effects are very similar to those of phenobarbital. It is currently hardly used in the treatment of epilepsy and if a barbiturate is to be used, phenobarbital is preferable.

OXCARBAZEPINE

Oxcarbazepine is a structural variant of carbamazepine with a similar efficacy, which is used an add-on drug for refractory partial seizures and as a first-line agent in previously untreated patients with tonic-clonic and partial seizures. Oxcarbazepine may exacerbate some types of generalized seizures particularly myoclonic seizures and absences. In addition to its antiepileptic action, oxcarbazepine is also used as an analgesic particularly in trigeminal neuralgia. Like carbamazepine, its putative mode of action is likely to be via the modulation of sodium channels. Oxcarbazepine is available in tablets and as an oral suspension: no other preparations are available. Its maintenance dose for adults usually ranges from 600 to 2400mg/day.

Oxcarbazepine shares many side effects with carbamazepine but overall oxcarbazepine is perceived as being better tolerated. Common side effects include nausea, dizziness, headache, drowsiness, agitation, lethargy, ataxia, impaired concentration, depression, tremor, hyponatremia, acne, alopecia, skin rash, and diplopia. Rare side effects include hepatitis, pancreatitis, arrhythmias, hypersensitivity reactions, thrombocytopenia, systemic lupus erythematosus, and Stevens-Johnson syndrome. Hyponatremia is more marked than with carbamazepine and occasionally leads to confusion and increase of seizures. Cross-sensitivity with carbamazepine for skin rashes is seen in about a third of patients. Oxcarbazepine should be started at a low dose and titrated up weekly to the initial target dose. However, if there are clinical needs and under supervision, oxcarbazepine can be started at the maintenance dose. It has less potential for pharmacokinetic interactions than carbamazepine but nevertheless, interactions occur, for instance, with oral contraceptives. Despite the fact that it has been available for almost two decades, not enough human exposure data has been accumulated to give it a clear bill of health with regard to teratogenicity.

RUFINAMIDE

Rufinamide is structurally distinct from other AEDs and has recently been given an orphan drug status for use in the Lennox-Gastaut syndrome both in the US and in Europe. Its mode of action is unknown. Its place in the antiepileptic armamentarium is, however, not yet clear. During studies the commonest adverse events were headache, dizziness, fatigue, somnolence, and nausea.

STIRIPENTOL

Stiripentol is an aromatic allylic alcohol unrelated to all other antiepileptic drugs which may be useful in the rare epileptic syndrome Severe Myoclonic Epilepsy of Infancy. It has an orphan drug indication for this condition. It does not seem to have any other indication in epilepsy. Its mechanism of action is unknown. Nausea and vomiting are often treatment-limiting side effects and it has also been associated with neutropenia and thrombocytopenia.

SULTHIAME

Sulthiame is a carbonic anhydrase inhibitor available in some countries as an adjunctive treatment for the treatment of both partial and generalized seizures: it is also said to be effective in Benign Rolandic Epilepsy. It is only available as tablets. The typical daily dose is 400-600mg. The commonest adverse events with this drug are nausea, paresthesias, headache, arthralgia, dizziness, and lethargy. It may rarely cause kidney failure and Stevens-Johnson syndrome. Its use should be avoided during pregnancy.

TIAGABINE

Tiagabine is a specific inhibitor of GABA uptake in glial cells and nerve terminals leading to a rise in extracellular GABA, and consequently increases GABA neurotransmission. It has a mild to moderate efficacy in the control of partial seizures. It has no indication in other seizure types and indeed is known to exacerbate generalized seizures. It is only available as tablets and the minimum effective dose seems to be 30mg/day. The commonest adverse events are central nervous system related and consist of sedation, tremor, headache, mental slowing, emotional lability, speech impairment, tiredness, depression, and dizziness. Rarely confusion, psychosis and leucopenia may occur. Increases in seizure frequency and episodes of non-convulsive status may also occur particularly when used in idiopathic generalized epilepsy. Enzyme inducers tend to accelerate the clearance of tiagabine and higher doses may be required if they are used concomitantly. Its use in pregnancy is not recommended.

TOPIRAMATE

Topiramate, a sulfamate-substituted monosaccharide, is chemically unrelated to other AEDs, and a number of putative mechanisms of action have been identified to account for its mode of action. It is a strong blocker of voltage-activated sodium channels and has a marked effect on GABA-A receptors. In addition, it blocks the kainate/AMPA type of glutamate receptors and is a weak inhibitor of carbonic anhydrase. It is not clear which one of these, if any, is relevant to its antiepileptic actions.

Topiramate is a broad spectrum drug for partial and secondarily generalized seizures. It is available only as tablets and sprinkle capsules. The usual dose range is between 75-400mg daily. Topiramate can cause predominantly neurological side effects, particularly at high dosage and if titrated too fast. These adverse effects include headache, sedation, impaired memory and concentration, speech disturbance, asthenia, anxiety, depression, sleep disorders, visual disturbances and confusion. Nausea, abdominal pain, dry mouth, taste disturbance, anorexia, weight loss, and paraesthesias may also occur. Topiramate may very rarely cause acute myopia with secondary angle-closure glaucoma which is reversible. To lessen the incidence of treatment limiting side effects, topiramate needs to be started at a low dose and it should be titrated up slowly. Topiramate is a weak inhibitor of carbonic anhydrase and as such is associated with an increased risk of renal stones; patients should be advised to increase fluid intake during treatment to decrease this risk. Enzyme inducers tend to accelerate the clearance of topiramate, and higher doses may be required if they are used concomitantly. Not enough human exposure data has been accumulated to give it a clear bill of health with regard to teratogenicity.

VALPROATE

Valproate is a branched chain fatty acid which is usually prescribed as the sodium salt in Europe. It is very effective in the treatment of all forms of idiopathic generalized epilepsies, and also in the treatment of secondarily generalized seizures. Its precise mode of action is unknown, although it may be in part due to an increase in brain GABA levels. Valproate is available orally in tablet, syrup and liquid form, and is also made as an intravenous preparation for patients temporarily unable to take the drug orally. Its use in status epilepticus is currently being evaluated.

The usual daily maintenance dose in adults ranges from 600-2500mg. Common side effects include tremor, behavioral disturbances, weight gain, thrombocytopenia, menstrual disturbances, ankle swelling, and usually minor loss of hair. Cognitive impairment is sometimes seen. Encephalopathy has been occasionally reported, possibly due to hyperammonemia, which is a common result of valproate therapy. Rare cases of fatal hepatotoxicity have occurred, especially in infants during polytherapy. Inhibition of platelet aggregation occurs but is not usually a problem except after surgery.

The use of valproate during pregnancy is associated with an increased risk of teratogenicity and there are concerns that it could also lead to increased educational needs in children exposed to it in utero, even when there is no malformation. Valproate should therefore be used cautiously in women of child-bearing potential. Valproate mildly inhibits the metabolism of other antiepileptic drugs which is rarely of clinical relevance except when prescribed with lamotrigine. Valproate inhibits the metabolism of lamotrigine, leading to greatly elevated plasma levels. The full pharmacological action of valproate may take several weeks to develop after steady-state concentrations have been reached. Valproate monitoring is not recommended as there is no relationship between clinical effects and the plasma concentration.

VIGABATRIN

Vigabatrin is an irreversible inhibitor of GABA-aminotransferase, the effect of which is to increase GABA levels in the CSF by up to 150% within days of starting treatment. In adults, it is used as a drug of last resort in refractory partial seizures. In pediatric practice, however, it is a first line drug for infantile spasms. Its use is currently limited by the occurrence of visual field defects in at least a third of patients on long-term therapy. Irreversible visual field defects, which may be asymptomatic in the early stages, can lead to blindness.
In view of this it seems prudent to limit its use to specialist centers in severe intractable cases.

ZONISAMIDE

Zonisamide, a sulfonamide, is a broad spectrum drug effective for partial seizures and for refractory generalized seizures, particularly myoclonic. It is available as capsules and no other preparations of the drug are currently available. Zonisamide maintenance dose for adults usually ranges from 150-500mg/day.

The common side effects of zonisamide include nausea, drowsiness, dizziness, irritability, depression, ataxia, speech disorder, impaired memory and attention, anorexia and weight loss, pyrexia, diplopia and skin rash. Less common effects include psychosis and hypokalemia. Rare side effects include hallucinations, suicidal ideation, amnesia, coma, neuroleptic malignant syndrome, heat stroke, hydronephrosis, renal impairment, blood disorders, rhabdomyolysis, impaired sweating, Stevens-Johnson syndrome, hepatitis and pancreatitis. Zonisamide is associated with an increased risk of kidney stones; patients should be advised to increase fluid intake during treatment to decrease this risk. Enzyme inducers tend to accelerate the clearance of zonisamide and higher doses may be required if they are used concomitantly. Despite the fact that it has been available for almost two decades, not enough human exposure data has been accumulated to give it a clear bill of health with regard to teratogenicity.

CHAPTER 8

THE SURGICAL TREATMENT OF EPILEPSY

8.1   When should surgical treatment be considered for epilepsy?

In some patients epilepsy is a symptom of a pathological process which can be identified by MRI scanning, while in others the nature of the underlying cause remains unknown despite investigation with currently available technology. In either instance, the seizures may be amenable to treatment by surgical means. If the underlying lesion is progressive (such as a tumor) or carries other inherent risks (such as the risk of hemorrhage from an arteriovenous malformation) the need for surgery may be determined by these considerations, regardless of seizure frequency. In patients without such a lesion, other criteria must be used to determine whether epilepsy surgery is appropriate.

The criteria for treating epilepsy by surgical means vary somewhat from center to center. There is wide agreement that *epilepsy should have been shown to be intractable to medical treatment before surgery is contemplated.* Such a trial of therapy should include treatment with at least two first-line drugs appropriate to the type of epilepsy separately, and with adequate compliance. Although it is often reasonable to try several different drugs alone or together over a period of time, the chance of a patient becoming seizure-free diminishes if control is not achieved with initial first-line drugs, and evaluation for surgery should not be unduly delayed while every possible combination of medication is tried. In a recent study carried out in Glasgow, Kwan and Brodie[1] found that among 470 previously untreated patients, 47% of patients became seizure-free during treatment with their first antiepileptic drug, and 14% became seizure-free during treatment with a second or third drug (3% required two AEDs to achieve seizure control). Only 11% of those in whom the first AED failed due to lack of efficacy rather than intolerable side effects subsequently became seizure-free.

Medication vs surgery

Epilepsy surgery is a major undertaking, and is only usually considered in patients with frequent seizures. Some centers suggest as a minimum an average of at least one seizure per week, but others consider patients with less frequent attacks,

Surgery is a major undertaking

if they are severe enough to significantly interfere with life style. Because of the physical and emotional strains of preoperative evaluation as well as the surgery itself, all patients should undergo psychological and psychiatric assessment, and only those patients with the resources to cope, either with surgery or the fact that surgery may not be helpful, should be offered further evaluation.

Some centers consider that patients with learning disabilities should not be considered for epilepsy surgery since they may have diffuse brain damage. However, recent studies have shown that patients with a lower IQ may derive benefit, either from resective surgery, or, for example, by the use of corpus callosotomy to treat frequent tonic or atonic attacks causing injury. Such patients should therefore receive consideration of operative measures if appropriate.

> People with LD and epilepsy may still benefit from surgery

8.2   What types of surgical treatment are available?

There are two main strategies for the surgical treatment of seizures. The first involves resective surgery, in which the aim of the *surgery is the removal of the epileptic focus itself.* Examples of this type of surgery are anterior temporal lobectomy (Figure 30), selective amygdalohippocampectomy (in which only the mesial temporal structures are removed), or resection of a frontal lobe or other lesion. At the other extreme of resective surgery, in patients in whom most or all of one hemisphere is abnormal, as in hemimegalencephaly or Rasmussen's encephalitis (an uncommon inflammatory condition causing seizures, progressive hemiparesis and intellectual deterioration), hemispherectomy (most commonly functional hemispherectomy) may be necessary. The other strategy for surgical treatment is to interrupt the pathways of seizure spread, thus isolating the epileptic focus from the rest of the brain to a greater or lesser extent. Examples of this type of surgery include section of the corpus callosum, and multiple subpial transection.

> Removing the epileptic focus

> Isolating the epileptic focus

Callosotomy was devised to prevent secondary generalization of seizures, and its chief indication is in the treatment of intractable generalized seizures, particularly atonic seizures. The procedure is sometimes carried out in two stages to try to avoid disconnection syndromes, in the hope that anterior callosotomy may provide satisfactory seizure control without the need for further surgery. Multiple subpial transection is a technique which relies on the fact that seizure spread in general occurs in a tangential manner through the cerebral cortex, while impulses controlling voluntary movement travel radially. In this operation, multiple cuts are made vertically in the cortex in an effort to isolate the epileptogenic area from the surrounding cortex. It may be helpful in the treatment of seizures arising in eloquent areas of the brain, such as the speech area or motor cortex.

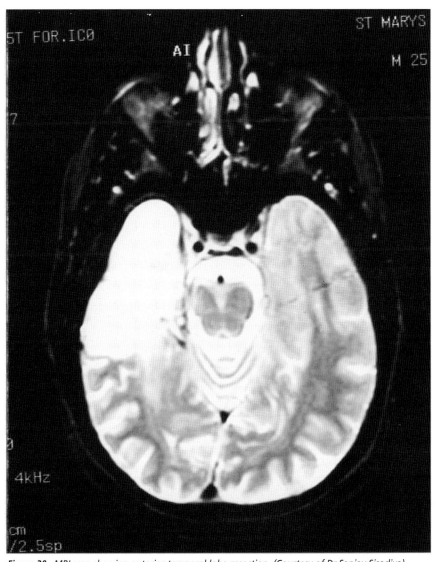

Figure 30. MRI scan showing anterior temporal lobe resection. (Courtesy of Dr Sanjay Sisodiya).

8.3   What determines the type and extent of surgery?

The type of surgery is dependent on the underlying lesion, its site and extent.
The most common type of surgery undertaken for epilepsy is temporal lobe surgery, usually anterior temporal resection (Figure 30), although selective amygdalohippocampectomy is used in some centers. Frontal lobe resection is carried out less commonly, and resection of the other lobes less often still, usually if a radiological lesion is present. Hemispherectomy is indicated in patients with infantile hemiplegia (or hemiplegia developing in childhood as a result of chronic encephalitis) and seizures arising from the diseased hemisphere.

Surgery is dependent on the lesion site and extent

In general, patients with multifocal or generalized epilepsy are not suitable for epilepsy surgery, except possibly corpus callosotomy. Until recently, patients in whom the epileptic focus was situated in a functionally eloquent area were also considered unsuitable: however, multiple subpial transection may occasionally be helpful in such cases.

8.4   What evaluation is necessary prior to carrying out surgery?

Pre-operative evaluation is largely directed towards the precise localization of the epileptic focus, and the need to ensure that resection will not compromise cognitive functions such as memory and speech.

Evaluation of the epileptic focus

Initial, non-invasive investigation includes interictal EEG studies during wakefulness and sleep, sometimes with sphenoidal or other electrodes suitable for recording from the anterior temporal region, magnetic resonance imaging (including volumetric assessment of the mesial temporal structures where appropriate), and neuropsychological and psychiatric assessment. If a structural lesion is identified radiologically and is concordant with the seizure pattern, EEG findings (both epileptic activity and background abnormalities), and neuropsychological findings, surgery may be possible without further investigation. If these conditions do not prevail, further investigation may be required, including prolonged EEG video monitoring, with reduction of antiepileptic drugs if necessary, to obtain an ictal EEG. A Wada test (intracarotid sodium amytal test), in which sodium amytal is injected into each carotid artery in turn and tests of speech and memory carried out, may be necessary to lateralize cognitive function and predict any

Maintaining cognitive functions

Non-invasive investigations

post-operative deficits, although in some centers this test has been abandoned and the decision to operate is taken on the basis of standard neurological testing and functional magnetic resonance imaging.

If the site of the seizure onset remains uncertain after these investigations, for example if there is discordance between the clinical seizure pattern and epileptic focus, or the apparent epileptic focus does not correspond to neuroradiological abnormalities, more invasive investigation with intracranial electrodes (such as depth electrodes or subdural electrodes) may be indicated. Further information as to the probable site of seizure onset may be obtained from functional imaging with SPET or PET scans.

Invasive investigations

8.5 How effective is surgery in the treatment of epilepsy?

The outcome of epilepsy surgery may be examined either in terms of seizure control alone, or with respect to its effect on wider issues, including psychiatric and social functioning.

Predicting long-term outcome

Seizures occurring in the immediate post-operative period are not necessarily predictive of long-term outcome, and are often excluded from the assessment of post-operative seizure control. Following surgery, many patients remain entirely seizure-free. Some patients continue to have seizures, but at a decreasing frequency, and their seizures may eventually "run down" and stop over a period of months or years. Still others are seizure-free after surgery, and for months or years thereafter, when a recurrence of their attacks occurs. Auras may continue to occur after surgery in some people, and if they do not progress to other seizures or interfere with daily life, such patients are usually considered to be "seizure-free". Based on these considerations, a classification of outcome following surgery has been devised by Engel (Table 7).

Freedom from seizures

The overall outcome with respect to seizure freedom depends on many factors, including the selection of patients for surgery, the underlying pathology (Figure 31), the length of follow-up, the center carrying out the surgery, and the policy regarding antiepileptic medication after surgery. It is common experience in reputable centers that at least 60% of patients become seizure-free after anterior temporal lobectomy, 45% after extratemporal resection, 75% after hemispherectomy, and 5% after corpus callosotomy (although a much larger percentage show some improvement).

I. **SEIZURE-FREE** (excluding early post-operative seizures)

   A. Completely seizure-free since surgery
   B. Aura only since surgery
   C. Some seizures after surgery, but seizure-free for at least 2 years
   D. Atypical generalized convulsion with antiepileptic drug withdrawal only

II. **RARE SEIZURES** ("almost seizure-free")

   A. Initially seizure-free but rare seizures now
   B. Rare seizures since surgery
   C. More than rare seizures after surgery, but rare seizures for at least 2 years
   D. Nocturnal seizures only, which cause no disability

III. **WORTHWHILE IMPROVEMENT**

   A. Worthwhile seizure reduction
   B. Prolonged seizure-free intervals amounting to greater than half the follow-up
       period, but not less than 2 years

IV. **NO WORTHWHILE IMPROVEMENT**

   A. Significant seizure reduction
   B. No appreciable change
   C. Seizures worse

(Engel J. (ed) Surgical Treatment of Epilepsy. New York: Raven Press 1993)

Table 7. Classification of outcome after epilepsy surgery.

With regard to psychosocial outcome after epilepsy surgery, a number of studies have shown some improvement in the majority of patients. The areas addressed in these studies have included interpersonal relationships, vocational adjustment, dependence, personal adjustment, and overall psychosocial functioning. However, such improvements are often limited to those patients becoming seizure-free or almost so. Even among patients experiencing good control of their seizures following surgery, a favorable psychosocial outcome is not guaranteed and an increased suicide rate has been reported after epilepsy surgery both in patients with a good and those with a poor result.

Psychosocial outcome

8.6   What are the risks of epilepsy surgery?

The hazards of epilepsy surgery embrace both the hazards of any neurosurgical procedure, and the specific hazards of the operation. Among the general risks of neurosurgery are those of death, hemorrhage, and infection. The complications of temporal lobectomy

The risks of surgical complications

include the possibility of hemiparesis (possibly due to manipulation of the middle cerebral artery), dysphasia, visual field defects, and damage to memory functions.

The risk of operative complications varies from center to center depending on the degree of experience and technical expertise of the surgeon. The overall mortality of temporal lobectomy is less than 0.5%, and the risk of permanent hemiparesis less than 1%. However, quadrantic field defect is common. This is not the case with selective amygdalohippocampectomy. Frontal lobe resection also carries a risk of motor and sensory defects and speech deficits.

In the past, classical (anatomic) hemispherectomies were complicated in as many as one third of instances by the development of superficial cerebral hemosiderosis, causing obstructive hydrocephalus and *Modified and functional* progressive neurological deficits. Such complications have been *hemispherectomies* largely prevented by the development of the procedures of modified hemispherectomy and functional hemispherectomy. In the former, the volume of the hemispheric cavity is reduced by sewing the dural flap to the falx and tentorium, thus creating a large extradural space. More commonly used now is the functional hemispherectomy, in which large parts of the frontal and occipital regions are left in situ, but disconnected from the rest of the brain. Mutism, akinesis and occasionally hemiparesis may be seen after corpus callosotomy, but are usually transient. Disconnection syndromes sometimes develop, particularly if a complete callosotomy is performed. Psychiatric complications may also occur following epilepsy surgery and an increased incidence of suicide has been reported even in patients becoming seizure-free.

VAGAL NERVE STIMULATION

For those patients in whom medical treatment is unsuccessful, and in whom surgery is not an option (for example, because the epileptogenic focus involves an eloquent area of the brain, or because the epilepsy is multifocal), vagal nerve stimulation may be a possibility. The technique involves the use of chronic intermittent electrical stimulation of the mid-cervical segment of the left vagus nerve, the stimulator wire being connected to a battery-powered pulse generator device implanted under the skin of the upper left chest. Typically stimulation is provided for 30 seconds every 5 minutes (though this can be varied), and additional stimuli can be provided by the use of a magnet to activate a switch (so that, for example, a stimulus can be provided when an aura is experienced, with the aim of trying to limit the further development of the seizure).

Vagal nerve stimulation is a palliative technique, and only provides complete control of seizures in a small number of patients (around 5%). Randomized controlled trials have shown a reduction of seizures by more than 50% in 23-31% of patients, although further improvement in seizure control may occur with time, and in case series, up to 71% of patients may respond. There is no clear consensus on the type of epilepsy most likely to respond.

Adverse effects include wound infection, and rarely, left vocal cord paralysis or lower facial weakness. Symptoms which may be experienced by patients at the time of stimulation include cough, hoarseness of the voice, throat pain, breathlessness, and headache.

Prognosis following epilepsy surgery	
PATHOLOGY	OUTCOME
Indolent glioma / DNT	Most favorable
Small vascular anomalies	
Hippocampal sclerosis	
Large / complicated AVMs	
Trauma	
Gross cortical dysplasia	
	Least favorable

Figure 31. Diagram to show prognosis following epilepsy surgery according to etiology. Reproduced with permission from Duncan JS, Fish DR, Shorvon SD. Clinical Epilepsy. Edinburgh, Churchill Livingstone, 1995.

CHAPTER 9

EPILEPSY IN WOMEN

9.1 Can seizures occurring in association with menstruation be helped by hormonal treatment?

Approximately two-thirds of women with epilepsy complain of an increase in seizures at the time of menstruation, but the term *catamenial epilepsy should technically be reserved for those patients whose seizures only occur immediately preceding or during menstruation* - probably about 5% of women with epilepsy. Several possible mechanisms have been put forward for this increase in seizure frequency, including the increase in the estrogen:progesterone ratio which occurs at this time, fluid and electrolyte imbalance; a fall in the level of antiepileptic drugs, and increased stress as a result of premenstrual tension.

> Menstruation and seizures

Various hormonal and other treatments have been used for catamenial epilepsy. Unfortunately they have been tried mostly in individual or small groups of patients (often those with intractable epilepsy which is not strictly catamenial) in an open-label, add-on manner, and the success of these maneuvers is thus difficult to judge, although it appears to be limited. Progesterone has been reported to cause a decrease in seizures in some women. Estrogens, on the other hand, have been shown to cause an increased susceptibility to seizures in animal models. However, the evidence that hormonal treatment significantly improves catamenial epilepsy is slight. The effect of diuretics appears to be similarly limited. Intermittent treatment in the perimenstrual period with adjunctive second-line antiepileptic drugs, such as acetazolamide or clobazam, has been advocated, and appears to help in some women.

> The effects of hormones as treatment

9.2 What advice should be given to people with epilepsy regarding contraception?

Those antiepileptic drugs (carbamazepine, oxcarbazepine, phenytoin, phenobarbital, and primidone) which cause induction of hepatic enzymes are associated with a decreased

> Decreased efficacy of oral contraceptives

efficacy of oral contraceptive agents, presumably as a result of increased hepatic metabolism of these agents (topiramate also reduces the efficacy of the combined oral contraceptive pill, but by a different mechanism). The hepatic enzyme-inducing drugs also increase production of sex hormone binding globulin, thus further reducing the amount of free progesterone. Patients taking the combined oral contraceptive pill (COC) in conjunction with any of these drugs should use a contraceptive pill with an increased estrogen content. In practice, a preparation containing at least 50 µg ethinyloestradiol is required (usually necessitating the use of two pills). "Tricycling", in which the pill is taken consecutively for 63 days, followed by a shortened (4-day) pill-free break, is also recommended. If breakthrough bleeding occurs, this should be taken as an indication that the agent may not provide adequate contraception, and a barrier method used in addition for the rest of the cycle. However, the absence of breakthrough bleeding does not guarantee the efficacy of the oral contraceptive pill.

Lamotrigine has also been reported to cause a decrease in levonorgestrel plasma concentrations and a minimal effect on ethinyloestradiol concentrations, but the practical effect of this on efficacy seems likely to be very small. However, it is also now known that the combined oral contraceptive pill may cause a clinically relevant decrease in the serum levels of lamotrigine, with an increase in trough lamotrigine serum concentrations in the "pill-free" period. Therefore, an increase in dosage of lamotrigine may be required when the COC is started by women with stable epilepsy treated with lamotrigine.

The efficacy of progesterone-only pills and progesterone implants may also be affected by these antiepileptic drugs, and their use is not recommended. Depot injections of medroxyprogesterone are unaffected by antiepileptic drugs. Intrauterine progesterone-only devices can also be used in women taking antiepileptic drugs.

9.3   What effect does epilepsy have on fertility?

Studies suggest that fertility in women with epilepsy is decreased in comparison with the general population, although the reasons for this are complex. It has been reported that people with epilepsy are more likely to remain single than the *Epilepsy's effect on fertility* general population, particularly if seizures develop early in life. The number of children born to married women is also lower than expected. Several studies have reported a reduction in sexual interest and activity in patients with epilepsy, particularly those with temporal lobe epilepsy.

It is likely that hormonal, social and other factors contribute to this decrease in fertility. The synthesis of sex hormone-binding globulin, which binds to testosterone and estrogen, is increased by phenytoin, carbamazepine and phenobarbital, thus reducing the concentration of free sex steroids. Enzyme induction by antiepileptic drugs may increase clearance of sex hormones. Increases in prolactin levels following seizures, particularly if frequent, can interfere with the hypothalamic-pituitary-gonadal axis and affect ovulation. Diseases of limbic structure or function may well affect hypothalamic function. Finally, psychological and social development may be affected by epilepsy, particularly in those patients with intractable seizures starting early in life.

9.4 What preconception counseling should be given to women with epilepsy?

The risk of teratogenesis is highest with polytherapy, and efforts should be made to reduce the number of drugs, to monotherapy if possible. In a few patients with good seizure control, a doubtful diagnosis, or those taking prophylactic medication, it may prove possible to withdraw antiepileptic drugs altogether.

Efforts to reduce drugs to monotherapy

However, if it is necessary to continue antiepileptic drugs, the patient should be advised of the risks but reassured that the chance of serious congenital malformation is low (See Section 9.7). *Folate supplementation (folic acid 5mg daily prior to pregnancy and for the first trimester) is recommended to try to minimize the risk of such malformations.*

9.5 What is the effect of pregnancy on epilepsy?

In some women, pregnancy appears to have little effect on seizure frequency or severity, and in some, there is an improvement in seizure control. *In about one third of women with epilepsy who become pregnant, however, a deterioration in seizure control is experienced.* This may be due to several causes, including a fall in antiepileptic drug levels associated with physiological changes in pregnancy, as described below, poor compliance with the levels of antiepileptic drugs due to concern about teratogenesis, and, in some patients, sleep deprivation. In the first trimester, the high estrogen:progesterone ratio may also play a part.

Deterioration in seizure control in some women

9.6   Is there any special monitoring which needs to be carried out during pregnancy?

During the second and third trimester of pregnancy there is an increase of plasma volume of approximately one third, causing a dilutional effect and a consequent decrease in the level of antiepileptic drugs. However, the increase in plasma volume is not the entire explanation for the change in drug levels. In the case of phenytoin, the decline is maximal in the first trimester, while the decrease in carbamazepine levels is maximal in the third trimester. The level of valproate also falls, but in a more constant manner. Blood levels of lamotrigine may fall to as low as 40% of the pre-pregnancy level in late pregnancy.

Monitoring during pregnancy

Other explanations for the alteration in plasma levels include changes in clearance, differences in plasma protein binding and, rarely, diminished absorption.

Because of these changes, it is advisable to see the patient regularly during pregnancy to keep a check on seizure control. *In patients who do not experience any change in seizure frequency, no specific changes are necessary.* In those with an increase in seizure frequency, it is helpful to monitor drug levels: because of the changes in plasma protein binding, free drug levels should be measured if possible. If a change in dosage of antiepileptic medication proves necessary, the pre-pregnancy dose of antiepileptic medication should be resumed at delivery. Particularly in women taking lamotrigine who are seizure-free and driving, it may be helpful to measure lamotrigine levels and adjust the dose appropriately.

Changes are not always necessary

9.7   What is the risk of congenital malformations in the babies of women with epilepsy?

The risk of fetal abnormalities in the general population is around 2-3%, but is higher in women taking antiepileptic drugs. The most common congenital malformations in the babies of mothers taking antiepileptic drugs are cleft lip or palate (accounting for almost one-third of the excess of malformations) and congenital heart defects, which occur in 1.5 to 2% of children, approximately three times that in the general population. Other major malformations include growth retardation, microcephaly, neural tube defects, and learning difficulties.

The risk of defects

In addition a number of more minor anomalies including hypertelorism, abnormalities of the epicanthal fold, short nose with broad nasal bridge, long upper lip, low set ears, hirsutism, low hairline, distal digital hypoplasia, ptosis and V-shaped eyebrows, may occur. *Congenital malformations may be associated with all the commonly-used antiepileptic drugs, and although various syndromes have been described for specific drugs, the overlap is wide.* It is recommended that folate therapy 5mg daily be given to all women with epilepsy before conception, and for the first trimester, to minimize the risks of congenital malformation.

Folate therapy can minimize the risks

The UK Epilepsy and Pregnancy Register[1] was set up to monitor the outcomes of pregnancies in women taking antiepileptic drugs. Carbamazepine and lamotrigine (at least in lower doses) appear to be two of the safer drugs, conferring a risk of teratogenicity of around 3%. The risk with valproate was approximately 6%. In general, the risk of teratogenicity appears to be greater when higher drug dosages are used, and in this study, the risk of abnormalities in patients taking high dose lamotrigine (greater than 200mg daily) approached that in women taking smaller doses of valproate (less than 1000mg daily). The teratogenic potential of many of the newer drugs, such as topiramate, levetiracetam, pregabalin, and tiagabine, is as yet unclear and such drugs should be used with caution in pregnancy.

Recently, concern has been raised about the possibility of extra educational needs in children exposed to AEDs during gestation particularly sodium valproate. The extent and causality of this has, however, not yet been fully elucidated.

9.8 Are there any other problems specific to mothers with epilepsy?

Several studies suggest that women with epilepsy are at greater risk of obstetric complications, including vaginal bleeding, anemia, hyperemesis gravidarum, and pre-eclampsia. Premature labor is more common than in women without epilepsy, and uterine contractions may be weak, so that intervention becomes necessary.

9.9 Should any particular problems be anticipated in the babies of mothers with epilepsy?

The majority of women with epilepsy give birth to normal healthy infants. Statistically there is a slight increase in

Normal, healthy infants

perinatal problems, with a tendency towards lower Apgar scores, and an increased risk of difficult labor, asphyxia, prematurity and low birth weight. The risks of teratogenesis are discussed in Question 9.7. The risk of neonatal jaundice may be decreased as a result of hepatic enzyme induction by AEDs.

9.10 Is it possible for patients taking antiepileptic drugs to breastfeed safely?

For the majority of women taking AEDs, breastfeeding may be undertaken without difficulty. AEDs are present in breast milk, at a concentration depending on the plasma protein binding (the more highly protein bound the drug, the lower the concentration in breast milk). Phenobarbital and primidone (which is metabolized to phenobarbital) sometimes cause problems with sedation, hypotonia and poor sucking, and occasionally it becomes necessary to stop breastfeeding on account of this. Jitteriness may occur in the baby on withdrawal of the drug. Benzodiazepines may also cause sedation in the infant. Hyperexcitability and poor sucking have occasionally been reported with ethosuximide. Women taking acetazolamide or topiramate are advised not to breastfeed.

Breastfeeding and antiepileptic drugs

9.11 What specific advice should be given to mothers with epilepsy who have young children?

Simple precautions should be taken by the mother with epilepsy when caring for her baby, particularly in the case of mothers having generalized tonic clonic seizures. Where there is a risk of dropping a baby, it is advisable to sit on floor cushions while feeding. For the same reason, washing and changing of the infant should take place on a waterproof mat placed on the floor. It is recommended that someone else should be present in the house when the baby is bathed. If it is necessary for a woman with epilepsy to carry her child up- or downstairs, she should use a carrycot to do so.

Care of babies and infants

CHAPTER 10

PSYCHIATRY AND EPILEPSY

10.1 What psychiatric disorders occur in people with epilepsy?

There are three main categories of psychiatric disorders occurring in people with epilepsy. First, *the underlying cerebral lesion responsible for the epilepsy may also predispose to psychiatric changes.* This may be seen, for example, in patients with frontal lobe tumors, and in those with Alzheimer's disease. People with diffuse brain damage, who often have learning disabilities, are also prone to both seizures and psychiatric disorders.

Predisposition to psychiatric changes

Secondly, *psychiatric disturbances may be directly associated with the seizures.* *Prior to seizures,* patients sometimes describe a prodrome in which they are tense, anxious, depressed or irritable [1]. The ictus itself may also be associated with various abnormal experiences, among them psychosensory, affective, cognitive, and psychomotor symptoms. Psychosensory symptoms include illusions and hallucinations involving any sensory modality: for example, objects may appear to be increased in size (macropsia) or distorted. The most common ictal affective symptom is fear, but anger may occasionally occur. Pleasant ictal affective symptoms are described but are rare. Cognitive disturbances during seizures include dysmnestic symptoms such as déjà vu or jamais vu, forced thinking and feelings of unreality. Clouding of consciousness, psychomotor symptoms and automatisms frequently occur during temporal lobe seizures. Automatisms often consist of chewing movements, fumbling with various objects or picking at clothes, and sometimes more complex activities such as undressing. They usually last only a few minutes, but on occasion may last longer.

Psychiatric disturbances and seizures

Cognitive disturbances

Occasionally ongoing epileptic activity may present as a confusional or obtunded state. This may occur in absence status, which occurs particularly in children, who appear confused, withdrawn and slow, sometimes alternating with a period of relative normality. A few cases of absence status occurring de novo in adulthood have also been reported. Complex partial status may present as a confused state, sometimes accompanied by automatisms and occasionally with psychotic features.

Post-ictal psychiatric disorders are also relatively common. The majority of people will be confused and have some impairment of consciousness immediately after a seizure. However, some then go on to have a period of relative lucency, usually lasting one to two days, followed by a "post-ictal psychosis" in which they experience hallucinations and delusions, often paranoid in type. Such psychoses, which are experienced on occasion by up to 18% of people with refractory epilepsy, may last for hours, days, or rarely even weeks. Treatment can be problematic as neuroleptic drugs tend to lower the seizure threshold: haloperidol, sulpiride or risperidone may be less likely to exacerbate seizures than some other drugs. Post-ictal psychoses not infrequently occur after a cluster of seizures, and it may be possible to avert them by aborting the cluster through the use of a benzodiazepine after the first seizure.

Confusion and impairment of consciousness

Finally, **psychiatric disorders which are not related to seizure activity can occur in people with epilepsy, particularly those with seizures of temporal lobe origin.** These include personality disorders, affective disorders and psychoses. The arguments about the existence of an "epileptic personality" are discussed below. Behavioral problems occur in some children with epilepsy, and are often linked to overprotection by their parents, so that they become socially isolated and are emotionally immature and dependent. A number of studies have shown depression to be common in patients with epilepsy, particularly those in whom the onset of the condition occurs late in life. Often this is reactive, though endogenous depression may also occur. Suicide is five times more common in people with epilepsy than in the general population, and in people with temporal lobe epilepsy, it is 25 times more common. Anxiety is also common in people with epilepsy.

Psychiatric disorders in people with epilepsy

Psychoses are more common in people with epilepsy, particularly those with associated neurological deficits, than in the general population. They particularly tend to occur in patients with long-standing, severe epilepsy, and are probably more prevalent in people with temporal lobe seizures, especially if a cerebral

Psychoses in people with epilepsy

malformation (such as hamartoma) is present. It has also been suggested that temporal lobe epilepsy associated with dysfunction of the left temporal lobe confers an increased risk of psychosis.

Interictal psychoses occurring in people with epilepsy may be intermittent or chronic. There may be affective, paranoid or schizophrenia-like symptoms; commonly occurring features are paranoid, mystical and grandiose delusions, feelings of passivity, and auditory hallucinations. There is often better preservation of personality and affect than in schizophrenia.

Acute psychosis may also occur in association with certain antiepileptic drugs, and has been reported, for example, with vigabatrin and ethosuximide. This seems to occur more frequently in people with previous psychiatric illness, those with associated neurological deficits, and those in whom seizures cease abruptly following introduction of the drug.

10.2 What is the prevalence of psychiatric disorders in people with epilepsy?

Assessment of the prevalence of psychiatric morbidity in people with epilepsy depends to a great extent on the definitions used, both with regard to epilepsy (whether, for example, people having seizures at any time in the past should be included, or only those with active epilepsy or receiving treatment), and with regard to the definition of "psychiatric disorder". Partly because of the unpredictability of seizures, epilepsy itself is often a considerable source of stress, and anxiety and depression are particularly common in people with epilepsy. Studies of psychiatric morbidity may also suffer from selection bias as a result of the choice of population under study, since it has been shown that people with epilepsy who also have psychiatric disorders are more likely to be referred to hospital. Thus hospital-based studies are likely to give misleadingly high results.

Overall, the prevalence of psychiatric disorders in people with epilepsy seems to be of the order of 30-40%, although it may be as high as 60% in people with neurological deficits in addition to epilepsy. Morbidity is also increased in people with temporal lobe seizure disorders. The prevalence of psychosis is much lower, with most studies giving figures of 1-3%, although some, mainly those studying hospital populations, give figures as high as 9%. People undergoing surgery for epilepsy

The prevalence of psychiatric disorders

(even where this is successful) may experience psychiatric morbidity afterwards, with 20-40% of people becoming transiently depressed. Psychosis may also rarely develop de novo after surgery for epilepsy.

10.3 What is "forced normalization"?

"Forced normalization"[2] is a term which was originally used by Landolt to describe a state in which certain patients with seizures showing epileptic activity on the EEG, at other times developed a psychotic disturbance associated with a lack of electroencephalographic epileptic activity. The term "alternative psychosis" is also used to describe this psychosis occurring in association with normalization of the EEG. Forced normalization may occur either during spontaneous remission of seizures or as a result of treatment with antiepileptic drugs. It is not limited to patients with temporal lobe epilepsy, having also been reported not infrequently in patients with generalized epilepsies, although its overall occurrence is rare (less than 1% of patients with epilepsy).

Forced normalization and alternative psychosis

10.4 Is there an "epileptic personality"?

Over the years there has been considerable debate as to whether an "epileptic personality" exists. Proponents of this view have suggested that certain characteristics are more commonly seen in people with epilepsy. Patients with temporal lobe epilepsy have been described as obsessional, circumstantial, "sticky", emotional, humorless, angry, suspicious, concrete, and with a preoccupation with religion and philosophy. Hyposexuality and hypergraphia have also been reported. Patients with juvenile myoclonic epilepsy, in contrast, have been described as having personality traits such as irresponsibility, quick temper, exaggeration and distractibility.

The debate over epileptic personalities

Although there are a number of factors which could explain an "epileptic personality", including the effect of medication, social isolation as a result of seizures, the stigma of epilepsy, parental overprotection, and underlying brain damage, **the existence of a personality disorder in patients with epilepsy in the absence of such factors remains unproved.**

10.5 Can the memory be affected by epilepsy?

Complaints of a poor memory are very common in people with epilepsy, particularly those with temporal lobe seizures. There

Complaints of a poor memory are common

are several factors which may be involved. In some instances, the underlying brain damage responsible for the epilepsy also causes memory impairment. In other patients, epileptic discharges occur frequently, and even though they may be insufficient to cause clinical seizures, they can interfere with memory function. Antiepileptic drugs are another possible cause of memory impairment, recognized with increasing frequency recently, although such problems are usually mild. A decline in memory may also be noted following surgery for epilepsy, particularly in people undergoing left temporal lobectomy.

Despite the fact that many people with epilepsy do complain of memory problems, *psychological testing often does not support the presence of a major memory disturbance.* This may be because the tests used are not sensitive to subtle abnormalities of everyday memory function, but it may be that some patients are unduly anxious about minor memory abnormalities which are common in the general population.

10.6 What are psychogenic non-epileptic seizures?

Psychogenic non-epileptic seizures (PNES) (also known as psychogenic seizures, hysterical seizures, pseudoseizures, or non-epileptic attack disorder (NEAD)) are *episodic disturbances which bear some resemblance to an epileptic seizure, but which do not have an epileptic cause.* PNES are common, being the diagnosis in up to 20% of patients thought to have intractable seizures. They not infrequently occur in addition to epileptic seizures in people with epilepsy, but in recent years have been recognized increasingly in people without an epileptic disorder.

PNES take many forms (for example convulsion, swoon, altered behavior), and have a variety of different causes. They may represent a misinterpretation of such symptoms as dizziness or anxiety (which may themselves be physiological or pathological). *Most commonly they have a psychological cause*, often an anxiety neurosis although occasionally they may occur in the context of a psychosis. Although PNES often take the form of a layman's image of an epileptic attack, they are usually not consciously simulated.

PNES have a psychological cause

Diagnosis may be difficult, particularly since some genuine epileptic seizures, especially those of frontal lobe origin, may have a bizarre appearance. However, it is often possible to

Distinguishing between epileptic and PNES

distinguish PNES on a clinical basis if one is witnessed, or recorded using prolonged EEG-video monitoring. The onset of PNES is often gradual, sometimes occurring in response to suggestion or the presence of others in the room. Initial cyanosis does not occur. Jerking of limbs is usually less rhythmical than is the case in epileptic seizures, often taking the form of wild asynchronous thrashing movements. Incontinence and injury may occur, but are less common than in epileptic seizures. Attempts to open the patient's eyes are often forcibly resisted.

Post-ictal drowsiness or confusion is uncommon, and the widespread slowing seen on EEG after a generalized tonic clonic seizure is usually absent. Measurement of serum prolactin levels in the post-ictal phase may sometimes be helpful in the distinction between convulsive PNES and generalized tonic clonic seizures, although it is less consistently useful in the diagnosis of more minor attacks. *PNES are refractory to antiepileptic medication, and a lack of response may be the first indication of this diagnosis in some patients.*

10.7   How should PNES be treated?

The treatment of PNES depends on the underlying cause, and may be complicated and difficult. If the diagnosis is the result of misinterpretation of symptoms, advice and reassurance may

Underlying issues of PNES

suffice. If the PNES are the result of more complex psychological problems, the underlying issues need to be examined closely and the help of a psychiatrist enlisted. It is rarely helpful in such cases to confront the patient with "putting on seizures" or reject him or her for the same reason; rather, a positive approach should be taken in which the attacks are recognized as a real problem, but treatment directed at the underlying disturbance.

CHAPTER 11

GENETIC COUNSELING

11.1 To what extent does genetic inheritance play a part in the development of epilepsy?

It has long been recognized that epilepsy has a genetic component, and that this is considerably greater in idiopathic than symptomatic epilepsy. A genetic predisposition is also indicated by the fact that many well recognized genetically-determined neurological disorders (such as tuberous sclerosis, fragile X syndrome, Angelman syndrome, and the mitochondrial encephalopathies) are associated with epilepsy.

It is likely that many forms of epilepsy have complex or multifactorial (polygenic) inheritance, in which there is an interaction between several loci and environmental factors. Examples of conditions with complex inheritance are benign epilepsy of childhood with centrotemporal spikes (BECCTS), and childhood absence epilepsy. Other patients have epilepsy related to chromosomal disorders (such as Down syndrome, and ring chromosome 20). In recent years considerable advances have also been made in the identification of Mendelian forms of epilepsy, where a single major locus accounts for the disease trait. Such conditions may have epilepsy as part of the phenotype (for example, tuberous sclerosis or Fragile X syndrome), or may be pure epilepsy syndromes.

> Genetic factors affecting epilepsy

Examples of primary Mendelian epilepsies include Autosomal Dominant Nocturnal Frontal Lobe Epilepsy (ADNFLE), Generalized Epilepsy with Febrile Seizures Plus (GEFS+), Severe Myoclonic Epilepsy of Infancy (SMEI), and Benign Familial Neonatal Convulsions.

ADNFLE is inherited as an autosomal dominant condition, in which frontal lobe seizures (sometimes with secondary generalization) occur in sleep, usually in clusters as the patient falls asleep, or shortly before awakening. More than one ADNFLE locus has been identified, with the genes coding for the nicotinic acetylcholine receptor.

GEFS+ was first described in Australia, the phenotype including the onset with multiple febrile seizures, followed by the development of afebrile seizures of various different types, including absences, myoclonus, tonic clonic and atonic seizures, and also partial seizures. It is inherited in an autosomal dominant pattern. A number of cases have been identified with mutations coding for voltage gated sodium channel subunits: others are associated with mutations in genes coding for the GABA-A receptor. Severe Myoclonic Epilepsy of Infancy (SMEI), which occurs in infants and is also characterized by the occurrence of febrile seizures followed by afebrile seizures, particularly atypical absences and myoclonus, but in which developmental delay then occurs, is also associated in a number of cases with the sodium channel gene SCN1A, and it has been suggested that this may represent the more severe end of the GEFS+ spectrum.

Benign Familial Neonatal Convulsions occur as an autosomal dominant condition in which seizures occur in the second or third day of life and stop within two to three weeks (though about 10% may develop epilepsy in later life). It is associated with mutations in potassium channel genes.

11.2   What is the risk of a patient with epilepsy having a child with epilepsy?

In view of the above, this clearly depends on the type of epilepsy. It is also affected by a number of other factors, for example, the sex of the parent with epilepsy (the risk being greater when the mother is affected), the age at which the parent developed epilepsy (the risk being greater if this was at a young age), the occurrence of epilepsy in the other parent or another sibling, and the presence of EEG abnormalities in the child at risk. Figure 32 summarizes these risks.
Genetic counseling may be helpful in quantifying the risks more precisely for an individual.

Quantifying the genetic risks

11.3   What is the chance of epilepsy developing in the sibling of a person with epilepsy?

Again, this depends on the type of epilepsy and other factors including age at onset and whether more than one family member is affected. Studies of children with generalized epilepsy have estimated the risk of epilepsy developing in siblings at about 4-9% (and of any non-febrile seizures at 6-12%), although almost 50% may show generalized spike and wave abnormalities on their EEG at some time. The risk is increased if a parent is also affected. For

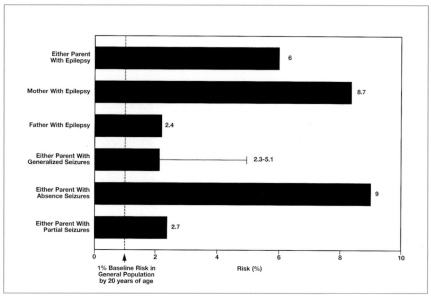

Figure 32. Diagram showing risk of an epileptic patient bearing a child with epilepsy. Reproduced with permission from: Hauser WA, Hesdorffer DC. Facts about Epilepsy. Landover, Epilepsy Foundation of America, 1990.

most patients with seizures of partial origin the risk of non-febrile seizures developing in siblings is about 3-5% by the age of 40 years. However, the chance of seizures developing is considerably greater (about 15%) in siblings of children with benign childhood epilepsy with centrotemporal spikes.

Development of epilepsy in siblings

11.4 What percentage of babies born to patients with epilepsy have significant congenital abnormalities?

Most estimates of the proportion of **babies having significant congenital malformations born to patients with epilepsy range from around 4 to 10%** although a few studies have found the rate to be as high as 16 to 18%. This compares with a malformation rate of about 2 to 3% in the general population.

Congenital malformations in babies

11.5 What are the principal causes of these?

There are several possible mechanisms. These include the facts that the epilepsy itself may be secondary to a genetic abnormality, and that anoxic or other damage may occur during seizures while the fetus is in utero. However, by far the majority of

Causes and risks of abnormalities

malformations are thought to be associated with the use of antiepileptic drugs by the mother during pregnancy, the "fetal antiepileptic drug syndrome". The risk is increased by the use of polytherapy, but the influence of serum drug concentrations on the risk of congenital anomalies remains controversial. There may be a slight increase in the risk of malformations in the children born to fathers taking antiepileptic therapy. Recent studies indicate that the risk of malformations is higher with some antiepileptic drugs than others. Thus the risk of a child having a malformation as a result of carbamazepine or lamotrigine therapy is of the order of 2-3%, whereas it is about 6% when valproate is taken in pregnancy. The risk is greater when the dose of medication taken in pregnancy is higher. There has also been a recent suggestion that the children of women taking valproate during pregnancy may have an increased risk of learning difficulties [1], though this has yet to be confirmed.

CHAPTER 12

WORK, LEISURE AND EPILEPSY

12.1   How does epilepsy affect a child's education?

In many countries recent government policies have encouraged a shift towards including people with disabilities in mainstream schooling, rather than advocating the provision of special schools. *In the UK the majority of children with epilepsy are now integrated into mainstream schools,* while most of those still being educated in special schools are there because of associated handicaps. Factors which may affect the educational performance of the child with epilepsy include such handicaps as the effect of medication, the effect of subclinical seizure discharges causing lapses in concentration or other cognitive impairment, and time off school as a result of epilepsy. Social isolation may also occur as a result of overprotection, problems caused by overindulgence, and low expectations by both parents and teachers. *The child should be encouraged to participate in almost all school activities and sports, with the possible exception of climbing.*

> Children with epilepsy in the mainstream classroom

12.2   How does epilepsy affect a person's prospects of employment?

Many studies have found an increased rate of unemployment or underemployment among people with epilepsy. This has been attributed to several factors. The seizures themselves may render certain types of employment (particularly where driving is involved) unsuitable; associated handicaps may also limit the choice of work. People with epilepsy may lack educational qualifications if they have missed a large amount of schooling, while parental overprotection may cause isolation and poor social adaptation. It seems probable, however, that the stigma of epilepsy has been responsible for a significant proportion of unemployment and underemployment, often because of a poor understanding about epilepsy or worries about public image, safety or insurance.

> Epilepsy in the workplace

12.3 Are there any jobs which cannot be performed by a person with epilepsy?

People with epilepsy are limited from holding posts in which driving is a necessity by the law prevailing in the particular country or state. The laws regarding the driving of passenger vehicles or heavy goods vehicles are usually stricter. Other areas of employment in which statutory barriers to the employment of people with epilepsy may be present are the police force, fire brigade, armed services and merchant navy, teaching, and the prison, coastguard and ambulance services. However, English law provides some protection for people with a disability (such as epilepsy), and requires the employer to take reasonable steps to avoid putting the person with disability at a disadvantage.

Potential job hazards

Types of work which could pose particular hazards for people with epilepsy include work with unguarded machinery, work near tanks of water or chemicals, and work with valuable fragile objects.

Where there are no statutory barriers, the type and severity of a person's epilepsy, the degree of seizure control, and the presence of associated handicaps are all important in assessing the suitability of a particular type of employment.

12.4 Does a person with epilepsy have to declare the condition when he or she applies for a job?

A dilemma may arise for the person with epilepsy applying for work if he feels that his seizures may present an obstacle to his obtaining the job. Failure to disclose the diagnosis can mean that the employer's insurance cover is invalidated. Provided that the epilepsy is disclosed and the employee is in a suitable job, most employers' insurance policies do not discriminate against disabled people. Where a prospective employee is required to complete a pre-employment health questionnaire, concealing the diagnosis may render the employee subject to dismissal and unable to claim that the dismissal was unfair at an industrial tribunal. However, to prevent the possibility of discrimination on account of one's health it is becoming increasingly common for such information to be disclosed only to the occupational health physician after recommendation for employment. The practices of individual companies may vary, but provided that the epilepsy does not constitute a bar to employment for safety reasons, it

Employment regulations for people with epilepsy

should usually only be necessary for the occupational health physician, and the employee's immediate supervisor in the case of active epilepsy, to know about the diagnosis.

12.5   Can people with epilepsy safely do shift work?

There has been little research into this aspect of employment. Issues of concern when people with epilepsy do shift work are that they should obtain adequate sleep, and that they should

Additional job safety concerns

take their medication regularly to avoid the risk of withdrawal seizures or seizures occurring during drowsiness. It has been reported that few problems have been encountered when these conditions have been met.

12.6   What restrictions on leisure activity should be placed on a person with epilepsy?

The risk of injury as a result of leisure activities depends partly on the type and frequency of seizures. *In general, the person with epilepsy should try to lead as normal and unrestricted a life as possible.*

Leading a normal life

Considerable psychological damage may occur as a result of overprotection. However, it is important to take simple precautions to try to minimize the risk of injury if seizures causing loss of consciousness should occur, and simple advice such as avoiding unguarded heights and not standing on the edge of station platforms, reservoirs and so on should be given. Participation in most sports is possible, even by people continuing to have seizures, although sub aqua diving, caving and contact sports such as wrestling and boxing should be avoided. *Swimming and riding are acceptable provided the person with epilepsy is accompanied by someone aware of the seizures who could help if necessary.*

12.7   What is the law regarding driving by people who have had seizures?

The law with respect to driving by people with seizures differs from country to country, and within the United States, from state to state. Most countries demand a period of seizure-freedom of one or two years before a license is granted,

Driving limitations

although in some the period is shorter or longer. The importance of seizure-type also varies; in some countries any type of seizure will cause loss of the driving license, while in others patients experiencing only simple partial seizures or myoclonic jerks are permitted to drive. The laws regarding the driving of heavy goods vehicles are usually stricter.

12.8 Does the law require a doctor to inform the licensing authority that his patient has epilepsy?

Again, this varies from country to country. In some the onus is on the patient, while in others, the doctor is responsible for informing the licensing authority about a diagnosis of epilepsy in one of his or her patients.

12.9 Does epilepsy have other legal implications?

Because of the nature of epilepsy, and in particular the fact that during both the ictal and post-ictal phases "automatic", subconscious, behavior may occur, it is occasionally claimed that crimes have been committed during the course of a seizure.

Important legal issues

Certain criteria should be fulfilled before an epileptic automatism can be held responsible. The person should be known to have epilepsy, there should be no premeditation, the offence should be inappropriate and out of character for the patient, and the patient should have impaired consciousness at the time of the offence, together with amnesia for the event. Although the prevalence of epilepsy among prisoners is considerably higher than in the general population, it is very rare for crimes to be committed during a seizure, and the increased prevalence can be explained on the basis of organic brain damage leading to impaired capacity, aggression and antisocial behavior.

CHAPTER 13

FREQUENTLY ASKED QUESTIONS BY PATIENTS

The following questions are those most commonly asked on the information service run by a voluntary organization for people with epilepsy. A brief answer is given in each case, together with the appropriate reference.

13.1 Where can I get some general information on epilepsy?

A list of websites of organizations able to provide such information is given in Appendix 2.

13.2 I have just been diagnosed as having epilepsy and want to know what I can or cannot do

People with epilepsy should try to lead as normal a life as possible. There are, however, some sensible precautions which should be taken to avoid injury in the case of seizures. These are discussed more fully in Chapter 12: they include swimming only when accompanied, and the avoidance of unguarded heights, water and fires. There are also restrictions on driving in patients with uncontrolled epilepsy, and certain professions are barred to people with epilepsy. It is important to advise each patient individually, taking into account the nature of his or her seizures.

Quality of life

13.3 I have just been diagnosed with epilepsy and want to know if I will have it for the rest of my life.

The majority (60-70%) of people developing seizures enter long-term remission, usually soon after starting medication, and in about 50% it is eventually possible for medication to be discontinued without recurrence of seizures. In a few people, especially those with such conditions as West syndrome and Lennox-Gastaut syndrome, seizures are more difficult to control (see Chapters 3 and 7).

Looking at the future

13.4 Who do I have to tell that I have epilepsy?

It is advisable for people with epilepsy, particularly if poorly controlled, to inform their immediate colleagues at work or teachers at school, so that appropriate measures may be taken in the event of seizures. It is also wise for patients to carry a card or wear a bracelet or medallion advising about their medical condition. Prospective employers may ask about medical conditions, and disclosure of epilepsy is advisable, even though this may cause some problems for persons seeking employment.

Informing the relevant people

13.5 Do the drugs that I take for my epilepsy have side effects?

All drugs have the potential to cause adverse effects in some people, as detailed in Chapter 7. However, if these do occur, they are often mild, and most people are able to take antiepileptic drugs with few if any problems.

Treatment questions

13.6 Is there any alternative to taking antiepileptic drugs?

People who have very mild or infrequent seizures, or only nocturnal attacks, may not need to take medication. Those having seizures only with known precipitants may also be able to manage by simply avoiding the triggering factors. However, in most people drug treatment is necessary, at least for a period of time. Surgery may be helpful in a small proportion of people who have not responded fully to antiepileptic drugs, but medication often needs to be continued afterwards.

13.7 Will the drugs that I take affect my having children?

There is a small increase in the risk of congenital abnormalities in the offspring of people with epilepsy, in part attributable to medication (see Chapter 9). However, the risk from uncontrolled seizures is greater in most women than the risk of continuing antiepileptic medication during pregnancy.

Concerns about pregnancy

13.8 My young daughter, who has epilepsy, has been told that she may not take part in such activities as swimming. Is this really necessary?

Most school activities, including swimming, can be undertaken by children with epilepsy, provided that supervision is

Children and sports

adequate. If seizures are uncontrolled, it is advised that the child avoids climbing activities (see Chapter 12).

13.9 How long do I have to surrender my driving licence if I have only minor seizures and do not lose consciousness during my seizures?

The laws governing driving vary in different countries, both with regard to the need to surrender the license if consciousness is not lost during seizures, and the length of time for which driving is not permitted. It is advisable to check with the appropriate authority in each case.

Driving and the law

13.10 How can I get in touch with other people who have epilepsy who could tell me about problems they may well have experienced and overcome?

The contact details from the national voluntary organizations for people with epilepsy can be obtained at the web site of the International Bureau for Epilepsy (IBE): www.ibe-epilepsy.org (please see appendix 2).

Epilepsy support groups

13.11 Can you give me any information about how to manage different types of seizures?

The acute management of generalized tonic clonic seizures is given in Chapter 7. The majority of seizures are self-limited, and no specific management is required apart from ensuring safety and reassuring the patient when the seizure is over.

Management of seizures

13.12 My husband and I would like to start a family, but I have epilepsy. Will our children develop epilepsy?

For the majority of people with epilepsy, the chance of a child developing epilepsy is very small (Chapter 11). It is slightly higher in some specific epilepsy syndromes, such as the generalized idiopathic epilepsies.

Inheritance of epilepsy

13.13 I have two children. The elder child did not have the whooping cough vaccine as my sister has epilepsy. Now I am being advised to have my younger one vaccinated. What should I do?

Although in the past it was advised that relatives of people with epilepsy should not be vaccinated, this advice has now been superseded (see Chapter 4).

Vaccination fears in children

13.14 I have had quite severe seizures for many years and the drugs do not seem to help. Could I be helped with surgery?

A proportion of people with seizures intractable to medical treatment may be helped with surgery. This is particularly the case for people with temporal lobe seizures. This is discussed in more detail in Chapter 8.

An alternative to medication

13.15 I had what doctors think were three seizures over the past six months but the EEG and MRI scan were normal. However, I am still being diagnosed as having epilepsy - why?

Although the EEG and MRI may show abnormalities in people with epilepsy, it is not at all uncommon for them to be normal. This is because epilepsy is an episodic disorder of neuronal function, i.e. in between attacks both the examination of the patient, and investigations may be unremarkable (see Chapter 6).

Investigation of seizures

APPENDIX 1

FURTHER READING

Arzimanoglou A, Guerrini R, Aicardi J. Aicardi's Epilepsy in Children (3rd edition). Lippincott Williams and Wilkins 2004.

Duncan JS, Panayiotopolous CP (eds). The typical absences and related epileptic syndromes. Edinburgh: Churchill Livingstone; 1994.

Duncan JS, Shorvon SD, Fish DR. Clinical Epilepsy. Edinburgh: Churchill Livingstone; 1995.

Hauser WA, Hesdorffer DH. Epilepsy: frequency, causes and consequences. New York: Demos Press, 1990.

Levy RH, Mattson R, Meldrum BS, Perucca E. Antiepileptic Drugs (5th edition). New York: Raven Press, 2002.

Luders HO, Comair, YG. Epilepsy Surgery (2nd edition). Philadelphia. Lippincott Williams and Wilkins, 2000.

Miller JW, Silbergeld DL. Epilepsy Surgery: principles and controversies. Taylor & Francis, 2006.

Panayiotopoulos CP. A clinical guide to epileptic syndromes and their treatment. Blaidon Medical Publishing, 2002.

Roger J, Bureau M, Dravet C et al (eds). Epileptic Syndromes in Infancy, Childhood and Adolescence (4th edition). John Libbey Eurotext, 2005.

Shorvon S, Perucca E, Fish D, Dodson WE. Treatment of Epilepsy (2nd edition): Blackwell Science Ltd 2004.

Shorvon SD. Status Epilepticus: clinical features and treatment in children and adults. Cambridge: University Press 1994.

Wyllie E (ed.). The treatment of epilepsy: Principles and practice (3rd edition). Lippincott Williams & Wilkins, 2001.

APPENDIX 2

EPILEPSY ORGANIZATIONS & OTHER USEFUL ADDRESSES

International Epilepsy Organizations & Epilepsy Resources in the Internet

INTERNATIONAL ORGANIZATIONS

The International League Against Epilepsy (ILAE) is an international organization for medical and paramedical professionals involved in the care of people with epilepsy. It has branches in over 90 countries. It headquarters are Brussels:

Avenue Marcel Thiry 204,
B-1200, Brussels, Belgium
Phone + 32 2 774 9547
Fax   + 32 2 774 9690
Website: www.ilae.epilepsy.org

Contact details for each of the countries chapters and officers can be obtained at the ILAE website.

The International Bureau for Epilepsy (IBE) is an international voluntary organization for people with epilepsy and their friends and carers. It has chapters and affiliated societies in many countries. Its main office is in Dublin:

11 Priory Hall, Stillorgan,
Dublin 18, Ireland
Phone: +353 1 210 8850
Fax: +353 1 210 8450
Website: www.ibe-epilepsy.org

Contact details for each of the individual countries chapters, affiliated societies and officers can be obtained at the IBE website.

EPILEPSY INFORMATION OF THE INTERNET

The internet provides a wealth of information on epilepsy for professionals, people with epilepsy and their friends and carers. This rather limited list provides some of the main reliable sites in English that provide information and resources on epilepsy.

Australia
- Epilepsy Action – Australia; www.epilepsy.org.au
- Epilepsy – Australia; www.epilepsyaustralia.org
- Epilepsy Foundation of Victoria; www.epinet.org.au

Canada
- Epilepsy Canada; www.epilepsy.ca
- Epilepsy Ontario; www.epilepsyontario.org
- Canadian Epilepsy Alliance; www.epilepsymatters.com

Ireland
- Brainwave - Irish Epilepsy Association; www.epilepsy.ie

New Zealand
- Epilepsy New Zealand; www.epilepsy.org.nz

South Africa
- Epilepsy South Africa; www.epilepsy.org.za

United States
- Epilepsy Foundation of America; www.epilepsyfoundation.org
- Citizens United for Research in Epilepsy; www.cureepilepsy.org
- Epilepsy.com; www.epilepsy.com

United Kingdom
- Epilepsy Action; www.epilepsy.org.uk
- Epilepsy Scotland; www.epilepsyscotland.org.uk
- Joint Epilepsy Council; www.jointepilepsycouncil.org.uk
- National Society for Epilepsy; www.epilepsynse.org.uk

REFERENCES

CHAPTER 2

1   Engel, J. A proposed diagnostic scheme for people with epileptic seizures and with epilepsy: Report of the ILAE Task Force on classification and terminology. Epilepsia 2001, 42: 796-803.

2   Commission on Classification and Terminology of the International League Against Epilepsy. Proposal for revised clinical and electroencephalographic classification of epileptic seizures. Epilepsia 1981, 22: 489-01.

3   Commission on Classification and Terminology of the International League Against Epilepsy. Proposal for revised classification of epilepsies and epileptic syndromes. Epilepsia 1989, 30: 389-399.

CHAPTER 3

1   Sander JW. The epidemiology of the Epilepsies revisited. Current Opinions in Neurology 2003; 16:165-170.

2   Kwan P, Sander JW. The natural history of epilepsy: an epidemiological view. Journal of Neurology, Neurosurgery and Psychiatry 2004; 75:1376-1381.

3   Hauser WA, Anderson VE, Loewenson RB, McRoberts SM. Seizure recurrence after a first unprovoked seizure. N Engl J Med 1982, 307: 522-528.

4   Hart YM, Sander JWAS, Johnson AL, Shorvon SD. The National General Practice Study of Epilepsy: recurrence after a first seizure. Lancet 1990, 336: 1271 - 1274.

5   Elwes RDC, Chesterman P, Reynolds EH. Prognosis after a first untreated tonic clonic seizure. Lancet 1985, ii: 752-753.

6   Hopkins A, Garman A, Clarke C. The first seizure in adult life: value of clinical features, electroencephalography, and computerised tomographic scanning in prediction of seizure recurrence. Lancet 1988, i: 721-726.

7   Gaitatzis A, Sander JW. The mortality of epilepsy revisited. Epileptic Disorders 2004; 6:3-15.

CHAPTER 6

1   Commission on Classification and Terminology of the International League Against Epilepsy. Proposal for revised clinical and electroencephalographic classification of epileptic seizures. Epilepsia 1981, 22: 489-01.

2   Commission on Classification and Terminology of the International League Against Epilepsy. Proposal for revised classification of epilepsies and epileptic syndromes. Epilepsia 1989, 30: 389-399.

3   Engel, J. A proposed diagnostic scheme for people with epileptic seizures and with epilepsy: Report of the ILAE Task Force on classification and terminology. Epilepsia 2001, 42: 796-803.

CHAPTER 7

1   Marson A, Jacoby A, Johnson A, Kim L, Gamble C, Chadwick D. Immediate versus deferred antiepileptic drug treatment for early epilepsy and single seizures: a randomised controlled trial. Lancet 2005, 365: 2007-2013.

2   Marson A, Al-Kharusi A, Alwaidh M, Appleton R, Baker G, Chadwick D, Cramp C, Cockerell O, Cooper P, Doughty J. The SANAD study of effectiveness of valproate, lamotrigine or topiramate for generalised and unclassifiable epilepsy: an unblended randomised controlled trial". Lancet 2007, 369: 1016-1026.

3   Marson A, Al-Kharusi A, Alwaidh M, Appleton R, Baker G, Chadwick D, Cramp C, Cockerell O, Cooper P, Doughty J. The SANAD study of effectiveness of carbamazepine, gabapentin, lamotrigine, oxcarbazepine, or topiramate for treatment of partial epilepsy: an unblended randomised controlled trial. Lancet 2007, 369: 1000-1015.

CHAPTER 8

1   Kwan P, Brodie MJ. Early identification of refractory epilepsy. N Engl J Med 2000, 342: 314-319.

CHAPTER 9

1   Morrow J, Russell A, Guthrie E, Parsons L, Robertson I, Waddell R, Irwin B, McGivern RC, Morrison PJ, Craig J. Malformation risks of antiepileptic drugs in pregnancy: A prospective study from the UK Epilepsy and Pregnancy Register. J Neurol Neurosurg Psychiatry 2006, 77: 193-198.

CHAPTER 10

1   Krishnamoorthy ES. Treatment of psychiatric disorders in epilepsy. In: The treatment of epilepsy (2nd Ed), Shorvon S, Perucca E, Fish D, Dodson E (Eds), Blackwell Science Ltd 2004: 255-261.

2   Trimble MR, Schmitz B. Forced normalisation and alternative psychoses of epilepsy. Wrightson Biomedical Publishing Ltd, 1998.

CHAPTER 11

1   Adab N, Jacoby A, Smith D, Chadwick D. Additional educational needs in children born to mothers with epilepsy. J Neurol Neurosurg Psychiatry 2001, 70: 15-21.

INDEX

F

G

H

I

J

L

M

QUESTIONS GUIDE

CHAPTER 5

CHAPTER 6

CHAPTER 7

CHAPTER 8

CHAPTER 9

CHAPTER 10

CHAPTER 11

CHAPTER 12

CHAPTER 13